EYE HEALTHCARE

A 90 YEAR HISTORY OF PROGRESS

[handwritten inscription and signature]

BY
PATRICK CONDON

Moyhill Publishing

© Copyright 2025 Patrick Condon

All rights reserved. No part of this publication may be reproduced, stored in a retrieval system, or transmitted, in any form or by any means, electronic, mechanical, photocopying, recording, or otherwise, without the written prior permission of the author.

The Moral Right of the author has been asserted.

First Published in 2025
ISBN 978-1-913529-22-2

A CIP catalogue record for this book is available from the British Library.

Moyhill Publishing
Unit 135393, PO Box 7169, Poole, BH15 9EL UK

Dedication

This book is dedicated to my parents Richard Augustine and Helen Agusta Condon, my wife, Ann, and our children Fiona, Richard, Edmund, and Jonathan

Contents

Introduction ... 1

Chapter 1 ... 5
Chapter 2 ... 15
Chapter 3 ... 19
Chapter 4 ... 25
Chapter 5 ... 35
Chapter 6 ... 41
Chapter 7 ... 53
Chapter 8 ... 67
Chapter 9 ... 73
Chapter 10 ... 95
Chapter 11 ... 107
Chapter 12 ... 117
Chapter 13 ... 135
Chapter 14 ... 143
Chapter 15 ... 151
Chapter 16 ... 167
Chapter 17 ... 175
Chapter 18 ... 183
Chapter 19 ... 197
Chapter 20 ... 209
Chapter 21 ... 213
Chapter 22 ... 223

Honoured Guest Awards ... 229
Jazz at the ESCRS ... 237
Acknowledgments ... 239
Appendix ... 240
Index ... 243

Introduction

It is hard to believe that in the main training centres for ophthalmology in Europe as late as 1930, the standard cataract operation techniques and instrumentation had hardly changed, since Daviel and von Graefe introduced their dramatic improvements almost two hundred years previously. The major significant advance came on the 29th of November 1949, 75 years ago, during removal of a cataract when Harold Ridley at St. Thomas' Hospital, London, inserted the first artificial lens implant. This was most probably the first of many major advances to occur in one aspect of eye healthcare that has had a major effect on the quality of life for individuals worldwide.

Since my father, Richard Augustine Condon started his ophthalmic training 90 years ago in the 1930s at the Royal Eye Hospital in London, and was a contemporary of Ridley, he was present at the Oxford Congress in 1951 when Ridley's results were heavily criticised by his colleagues at Moorfields Eye Hospital. This book is a record of the major advances in eye healthcare experienced by both of us as ophthalmic surgeons actively involved with the people that we met during that period and the lasting effect it has made in bringing eye healthcare to the communities we served.

Eye healthcare encompasses the medical science advocated in the practice of ophthalmology which includes not only the medical and surgical aspects of the specialty, but also the science of visual optics, closely related to the gift of sight. Whereas the main object in the practice of ophthalmology, concerns the diagnosis and treatment of diseases affecting sight, the delivery of eye healthcare must inevitably involve itself in aspects of preventative care. As prevention is primarily a community based activity with wider social implications, it can easily be ignored as being beyond the control of the eye healthcare provider. In the development of an eye healthcare service, there are many aspects which will be referred to in this book recounting the challenges faced by my father and his fellow colleagues, as well as myself and my colleagues down through the years. As a result of constant advocating by the public and our professional societies, what we have achieved to date, is now regarded as the norm.

When it comes to the changes in eye healthcare that we have witnessed in Europe, there is no doubt, that the transformation in cataract surgery has been a major advance in the restoration of sight and the quality of life for all. The rapid restoration of sight in a patient of my father, who after removal of a cataract, had an artificial lens implanted in the late 1950s by him, was probably one of the first of many to have benefited from lens implantation, and signalled a seismic change in eye healthcare in Ireland at the time.

In writing a book concerning the delivery of eyecare, one is confronted with a myriad of issues involving firstly, the quality of training in the specialty for medical graduates, aspects of community-based medicine, hospital management, and government resources, which invariably eclipse the actual challenges the ophthalmologist must deal with at the coalface. The ophthalmologist of today must also deal with the rapidly evolving technology involved in eyecare and the incredible number of new skills to be acquired using these technologies. With all the developments in ophthalmology in the last hundred years, and with a personal involvement until relatively recently, I feel it is important to look back at some of the major medical and social advances that have been made during that period, and which have transformed our eye health-care in Ireland and the UK.

All profits from the sale of this book will go to the Ridley Eye Foundation (REF), whose mission it is to provide funding for the sustainable delivery of surgery for the needy people of the developing world who suffer from cataract blindness. The focus is currently treating poor patients who live in the foothills of the Himalayan mountains in Nepal above 2000 m. REF aims to become the UK's leading high altitude cataract surgical charity and by 2027 to be providing up to 30 surgical camps per year extending its services to all five Himalayan provinces by 2032.

Richard Augustin Condon:

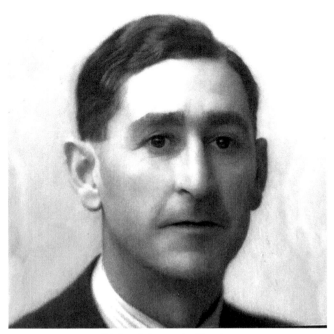

Richard Augustin Condon

The story begins with my father, Richard Condon, who was born on the 19th August 1897, the third child and first son to William and Mary Elizabeth Condon (O'Connell) in Shronell House, Lattin, County Tipperary. Richard's father, my grandfather, William, was a general medical practitioner and dispensary doctor for Lattin and surrounding areas of Belleville, Emly, and Knocklong. Following a secondary education at Rockwell College in Co. Tipperary, he was accepted into medical school and qualified at the National University of Ireland (NUI), University College Dublin (UCD) in 1921. After a year as an intern at the Richmond Hospital in Dublin, he emigrated to the UK spending the next few years as a senior house officer working in geriatrics and infectious diseases, ending up in general practice in Oldham, north England for 5 years.

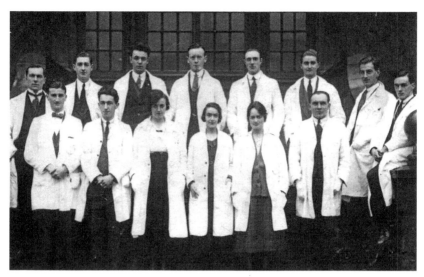

1921 Final Medicine NUI

Chapter 1
Becoming an Ophthalmologist – 1930's

Whatever possessed Richard to return to London to apply for a post in ophthalmology is not known, but after six years in general practice and considerable experience in treating mental illness and infectious diseases, it was obvious that a surgical specialty was more in his line. The two main centres for training in ophthalmology in London were Moorfields Eye Hospital, City Road, North London, and the Royal Eye Hospital at St. George's Circus in Southeast London. Moorfields Eye Hospital, originally known as the hospital for Curing Diseases of the Eye and Ear, was founded in 1805, moving to Lower Moorfields, close to nearby Liverpool Street station in 1822, remaining there ever since to serve the population north of the Thames. At the time, Sir Stewart

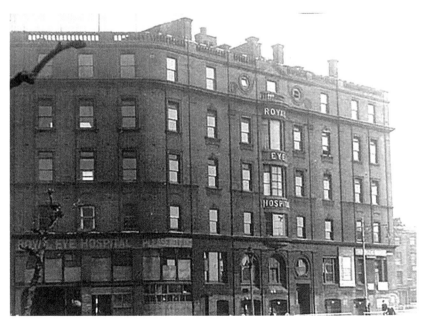

Royal Eye Hospital, Southwark, SE 11

Duke Elder, who worked at the Institute of Ophthalmology in Judd Street and allied to Moorefield's, was beginning to write his twelve volumes of "Systems in Ophthalmology" textbooks which attracted aspiring ophthalmologists wishing to work there.

While St. Thomas' Hospital was built in 1886 to serve the people of London south of the river Thames, the Royal Eye Hospital originally known as the Royal South London Ophthalmic Hospital, was founded in 1857 at St. George's Circus, just down the road from Waterloo railway station where it remained and provided ophthalmic services for the south London area extending right down to the Surrey border, where the Royal Sussex Eye Hospital built around the same time, took over the eyecare for Kent, Surrey and Sussex in the Brighton area.

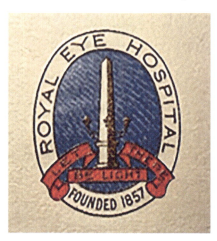

Royal Eye Hospital, London

Following his application to join the training program in ophthalmology in 1931, Richard was accepted and appointed as a

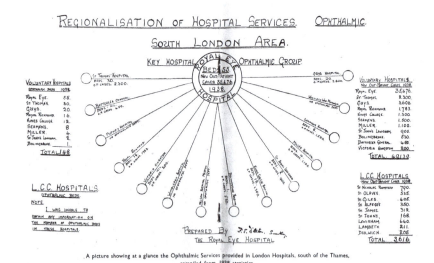

Royal Eye Hospital Service Area

ROYAL EYE HOSPITAL

[KING'S COLLEGE HOSPITAL GROUP]

ST. GEORGE'S CIRCUS, S.E.1

LECTURES
AUTUMN TERM, 1951

ANATOMY, PHYSIOLOGY AND OPTICS

By arrangement with the Royal College of Surgeons and the Institute of Ophthalmology the systematic lectures on Anatomy and Physiology will be given at the Royal College of Surgeons by the Staff of the College. Applications may be made direct to the College or to the Secretary, The Royal Eye Hospital. The following special lectures will be given at the Royal Eye Hospital.

Lecture	Lecturer	Date	Time
MALCOLM McHARDY LECTURE — Selected Features of Applied Anatomy of the Orbit	Prof. Thomas Nicol, M.D., D.Sc., F.R.C.S.	Monday, November 26th	5.30 p.m.
LAURENCE-HOLTHOUSE LECTURE — The Endocrines and the Eye	Dr. C. A. Keele, M.D., M.R.C.P.	Friday, November 30th	5.30 p.m.
ARTHUR D. GRIFFITH LECTURE — The Optical Principles of Ophthalmoscopy and Retinoscopy	Mr. J. F. P. Deller, M.A., B.Sc.	Wednesday, October 10th	5.30 p.m.

CLINICAL OPHTHALMOLOGY

LECTURES ON SURGERY OF THE EYE

Subject	Lecturer	Date	Time
Ophthalmic Injuries	Mr. T. M. Tyrrell	Tuesday, October 16th	5.0 p.m.
Plastic Operations and Orbital Surgery	Miss J. M. Dollar	Thursday, October 18th	5.30 p.m.
Detachment of the Retina	Mr. Arnold Sorsby	Monday, October 22nd	5.0 p.m.
Glaucoma	Mr. L. H. Savin	Wednesday, October 24th	5.30 p.m.
Squint	Mr. A. J. Cameron	Friday, October 26th	4.30 p.m.
Points in the selection, testing, maintenance, and use of ophthalmic instruments	Mr. A. J. Cameron	Friday, November 2nd	4.30 p.m.
Lacrimal Sac and Ducts	Mr. R. P. Crick	Wednesday, November 7th	5.30 p.m.
Cataract	Miss M. Savory	Friday, November 9th	5.0 p.m.

OTHER LECTURES

Subject	Lecturer	Date	Time
Congenital Fundus Lesions	Mr. Arnold Sorsby	Monday, October 29th	5.0 p.m.
Anaesthetics in Ocular Surgery	Dr. J. H. Willis	Thursday, November 1st	5.30 p.m.
Abiotrophic Fundus Lesions	Mr. Arnold Sorsby	Monday, November 5th	5.0 p.m.
Bacteriology of the Eye	Dr. A. C. Cunliffe	Tuesday, November 6th	5.0 p.m.
Inflammatory Affections of the Fundus	Mr. Arnold Sorsby	Monday, November 12th	5.0 p.m.
The Facies in Disease	Mr. L. H. Savin	Wednesday, November 14th	5.30 p.m.
Post-operative complications and their management	Miss J. M. Dollar	Thursday, November 15th	5.30 p.m.
The Newer Antibiotics	Mr. Arnold Sorsby	Monday, November 19th	5.0 p.m.
Fundus Appearance in Vascular Disease	Mr. R. P. Crick	Wednesday, November 28th	5.30 p.m.
Demyelinating Diseases in Ocular Practice	Dr. S. Nevin	Thursday, November 29th	5.0 p.m.
The Science and Art of Refraction	Dr. T. H. Whittington	Mondays, December 3rd, 10th, 17th, 31st, January 7th, 14th, and 21st	5.0 p.m.
Recent Applications of Physiology and Pharmacology to Ocular Therapeutics	Miss M. Savory	Friday, December 7th	5.0 p.m.
Pseudoglioma	Mr. R. P. Crick	Wednesday, December 12th	5.30 p.m.
Ocular Complications of Arthritic Disease	Mr. L. H. Savin	Wednesday, January 2nd	5.30 p.m.
Ptosis	Dr. T. H. Whittington	Monday, January 28th	5.0 p.m.

LECTURES TO NURSES AND OPHTHALMIC AUXILIARIES

| | Miss Iris Kane | Tuesdays, November 13th, 20th, 27th | 5.30 p.m. |

DEMONSTRATIONS

Pathological Specimens	Mr. R. P. Crick	Tuesday, January 15th	5.0 p.m.
Ward Round (Eye Unit, Lambeth Hospital)	Mr. Arnold Sorsby	Mondays, October 1st to December 17th	2.0 p.m.

REVISION CLASSES

Date	Lecturer	Time	Date	Lecturer	Time
Wednesday, December 5th	Mr. H. N. Reed	5.0 p.m.	Wednesday, January 16th	Mr. H. N. Reed	5.0 p.m.
Wednesday, December 19th	Mr. H. N. Reed	5.0 p.m.	Thursday, January 17th	Miss M. Savory	5.30 p.m.
Thursday, January 3rd	Miss J. M. Dollar	5.30 p.m.	Tuesday, January 22nd	Mr. T. M. Tyrrell	5.0 p.m.
Tuesday, January 8th	Mr. T. M. Tyrrell	5.0 p.m.	Wednesday, January 23rd	Mr. L. H. Savin	5.30 p.m.
Wednesday, January 9th	Mr. L. H. Savin	5.30 p.m.	Tuesday, January 29th	Mr. T. M. Tyrrell	5.0 p.m.
Thursday, January 10th	Miss M. Savory	5.30 p.m.	Wednesday, January 30th	Mr. H. N. Reed	5.0 p.m.

The Lectures at the hospital are open to both postgraduate and undergraduate students. Attendance at Demonstrations and Revision Classes is limited and tickets of admission should be obtained from the Secretary.

Royal Eye Hospital, Lecture Programme Autumn 1951

junior house officer at the Royal Eye Hospital, in Southwark, South London. The senior consultants attending at the hospital were, Arthur Griffith, Lewis Savin, TW Letchworth, Myles Bickerton, AF McCollum, and Arnold Sorsby, all of whom were eminent ophthalmic surgeons experienced in the various subspecialties of ophthalmology.

Arnold Sorsby, FRCS, MD (1900–1980) was of émigré stock, being born in Poland (Białystok) on 10th June 1900, a son of Jacob Sourasky and his wife Elka (Slomianesky). His surname was changed by deed poll about 1930 to Sorsby. After attending a community school in Antwerp, his education continued at the Central High School in Leeds. After qualifying in medicine at Leeds University at the age of 21, he received the FRCS and MD at 28 and 29 years of age respectively and was appointed as a surgeon to the to the London Jewish Hospital, the Hampstead General Hospital, and the West End Hospital for Nervous Diseases. At the age of 31, he was appointed to the Royal Eye Hospital as a consultant ophthalmic surgeon where Richard Condon worked with him in the outpatient clinics and operating theatres. He subsequently became Dean of the medical school from 1934 to 1938 and from 1934 to 1966, was Research Professor of Ophthalmology at the Royal College of Surgeons and the Royal Eye.

The Evolution of Cataract Surgery:

In 1747, having used the historic technique of couching to treat cataract for several years, Dr. Daviel in France described his new operation, whereby the surgeon sitting in front of the patient, would open the eye using a sharp knife with a stab incision, enlarge the incision with a scissors and removing the cataract from within the lens, leaving the residual part or the outer skin of the lens intact. This was called the extracapsular cataract procedure using an ab externo (from outside) approach. This continued until Albrecht von Graefe (1828–1870) changed the technique with the use of his specially designed cataract knife which was used by the surgeon sitting at the top of the table with the patient lying down in the face up position. The Graefe knife was then inserted from the side in the 3 or 9 o'clock position of the cornea (depending on Rt or Lt eye), passed internally across the anterior chamber of the eye in front of the pupil, to exit from the opposite corner, followed by an upper cutting sawing motion to exit the eye in the 12 o'clock position. This ab interno (from inside) incision, cutting from the inside of the eye upwards, which had to be done swiftly so as not to lose the anterior chamber depth and risk snagging the pupil, took a great deal of skill especially with poor anaesthesia. An opening was then made in the capsule of the lens, called the capsulotomy and the nucleus containing the cataract was expressed from the eye with gentle pressure from below externally while gently washing out the remnants of the lens with an irrigating fluid. After the operation, the patient had to lie immobile for several days with both eyes bandaged until the wound had closed completely. At the time, this was the standard procedure used by surgeons at the Royal Eye Hospital, but with the addition of a 5-0 black or virgin silk suture to close the incision for faster post operative recovery.

Ophthalmology Training in the 1930s:

Being a total beginner to ophthalmology, it took a considerable amount of time for Richard to learn the ropes, but month by month with his experience of dealing with patients, he soon learned how to examine the eye and the basic treatments while working with the various consultants. It was not long before he began picking up the minor operation techniques such as lacrimal washouts, removal of chalazions, corneal foreign bodies and other minor lid surgical skills before moving on, as a registrar, to where he could then participate in more major procedures. During his time at the Royal Eye, he attended the clinics and operated with all the consultants, acquiring the surgical and technical skills required to use the special equipment needed to examine patients with eye diseases. In this capacity, because the Royal Eye Hospital was the major ophthalmic hospital south of the Thames, with its emergency department being continually busy in dealing with up to 100 patients a day and on duty at night, his experience of dealing with emergencies became part of his training. Another part of his duties included working with the chief technician, Mr. Stevens in the laboratory where he studied basic eye pathology, bacterial infections and preparing specimens. Having become completely fascinated with ophthalmology, he began studying the basics sciences of that specialty, such as optics, anatomy, physiology, and diseases of the eye in preparation for the diploma of ophthalmology examination and initiated a series of lectures in the subjects for postgraduates taking the examinations.

Higher Qualifications and Professional Experience:

In 1932, Richard received the Diploma in Ophthalmology (DO Oxford) followed by the Diploma in Ophthalmology Medicine and Surgery RCS London (DOMS) the following year. Having achieved excellent training under the supervision of some of the best ophthalmologists in London, Richard was now beginning to take up his position of seniority and to diversify his clinical experience beginning as Chief Clinical Assistant at the Royal Eye Hospital, and was appointed to sessions at the Western Ophthalmic Hospital, the Royal Waterloo Hospital, King's College Hospital as well as being an outpatient officer to Mr. Foster Moore, a senior surgeon at the Royal London Ophthalmic Hospital (Moorefield).

As Richard considered himself fully trained surgically and with Dr. H. Whittington looking for a surgical partner at the time, Richard launched himself into private practice at 146, Harley St., London in partnership with him. During his period working with Dr. Whittington, Richard carried out many of the surgical procedures required for the practice. Like all surgeons at the time,

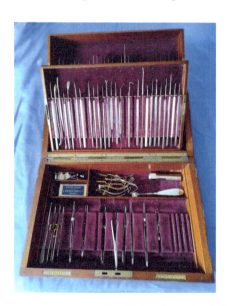
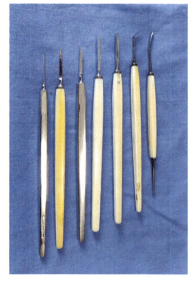

Dr. Richard Condon's Surgical Instruments

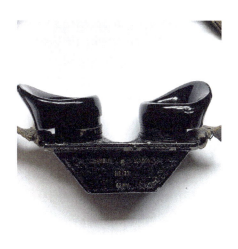

Dr. Richard Condon's Binocular Loupes

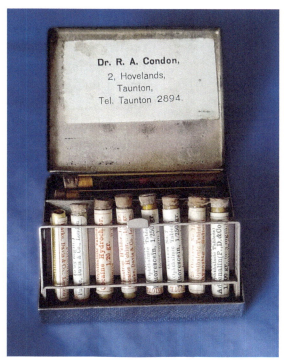

Medicines pillbox used by general practitioners

he carried his own extensive range of surgical instruments with him, making sure to always have a spare sharp Graefe knife to guarantee perfect cataract incisions and loupes for improved magnification during surgery.

As evidenced by the green plaque placed by the London City

of Westminster outside 146, Harley St., in recent years, Lionel Logue, speech therapist to the Duke of York, before becoming King George VI, practiced in the building from 1922 to 1953. It is highly likely that the King was being treated in the same building as Richard at the time.

It was also at this time of his life, that he was promoted to Surgeon Lieutenant Commander (Ophthalmology) to the Royal Naval Volunteer Reserve Force.

Helen Augusta Condon (Dransfield) 1911–1995:

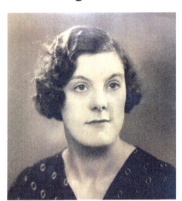

Ms. Helen Augusta Dransfield

My mother, Helen Agusta Condon was born in Oldham, Lancashire in 1911, the second child of Frank and Jane Dransfield (Ogden). My grandfather, Frank Dransfield, was born in 1887 in Denshaw (Parish of Saddleworth), a neighbouring town to Oldham but situated in Yorkshire just over the border from Lancashire. For a period of his life, Frank was managing director of a well-known brickworks

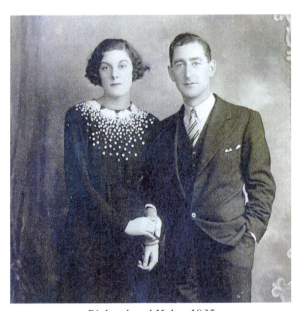

Richard and Helen 1935

and clay pipe manufacturing company owned by Thomas Mellodew & Co at Littleborough, near Rochdale. On contracting tuberculosis, he and the family moved to live in Wellesbourne, Warwickshire while Helen was designated to take over the management and running of the company at 21 years of age.

Meanwhile Richard while still working as a clinical assistant in the above London hospitals, found time to renew his friendship with Helen Dransfield, that had been initiated, while he had worked in general practice in the Oldham region. Helen was visited by Richard in the family home of her parents who lived in the White House in Wellesbourne. Having decided that they were for each other, Richard, age 37, and Helen age 23 were married on 21st March 1935, at St. Gregory's Roman Catholic Church in Stratford-upon-Avon, Warwickshire, England. A year later in 1936, Frank Dransfield passed away and was buried in the church grounds at Wellesbourne, a short distance from the White House where he and his wife had lived.

Chapter 2
Change of Direction 1935–1943

Having achieved a very successful career in ophthalmology in London, and wanting to have a family, my parents decided to set up house out of the busy London ambiance and moved to a terraced house at 2, Hovelands in Taunton, Devon in 1935. Initially my father set himself up as a general practitioner working from our house and employing my mother as an assistant pharmacist, making up and dispensing routine medications for the patients which was the norm at that time. During this period, Richard approached the West of England Eye Infirmary in Exeter and subsequently worked as an honorary ophthalmic surgeon there. He was also appointed to the Taunton and Somerset Hospital in Taunton as visiting ophthalmic surgeon and carried out eye clinics in some of the other hospitals in the Devon and Somerset areas with some private practice in conjunction with a friendly ophthalmologist, Dr. Nesus.

Condon Family:

I was born on the 10th April 1936, at a nursing home in Exeter and was followed by my brother, David, born a year later but who died shortly after birth, and which gave my mother great grief. On 15th April 1938, my sister Elizabeth was born followed by Diana in 1939. From the outbreak of war in September 1939, Hitler began his offensive against England which involved regular nightly air raid attacks on London and the major cities of England. With the increasing intensity and escalation of the war from 1939, it was decided that my mother and my two sisters, Elizabeth and Diana and I should be sent to Ireland for our safety, and in 1941, the family arrived in Dun Laoghaire from the Mail boat and settled in rented accommodation in Killiney, Co. Dublin. Meanwhile, my father, who remained in England, continued to work in the

Devon /Somerset areas, fulfilling his naval reserve commitment and spending some time on HMS Hood, the most modern warship of the Royal Navy. Being concerned about my education, he requested my mother to source a school run by the Christian Brothers which turned out to be the Irish speaking CBS Synge St. in central Dublin.

From 1941 to 1943, while my father continued to work as an ophthalmologist in the Devon/Somerset area, he still managed to return to the family at frequent intervals until he developed a period of illness, the gravity of which necessitated him informing his employers at the hospitals and clinics. This was greeted by surprise at the time, followed by an outpouring of concern from individuals, colleagues in the Devon/Somerset areas, and local government organizations who commended him for the extent of service that had provided for the people in that area and wished him well in his recovery. It was during this time that my youngest sister Teresa was born in Dublin on 15th May 1943.

RAC Return to Ireland–1943:

Following Teresa's birth, my father finally resigned completely and returned to Ireland to live with our family. There then followed a period in which to decide where we were eventually going to settle and being a Tipperary man, my parents finally decided to move to Clonmel in County Tipperary. We acquired accommodation at Oakville, a large lovely old house in the middle of Clonmel town situated at the end of Queen Street. In his effort to seek work as an ophthalmologist, he contacted some of his colleagues who qualified with him in Dublin many years previously. Many of them were scattered all over the country in various posts. One of these was Mr. Jock O'Halloran, a general surgeon in Roscommon Hospital, who indicated that there was a shortage of ophthalmologists in his area and organized for my father to travel to Roscommon to do clinics there. At this stage, he abandoned his bicycle which he had been using up to this and bought a Model T Ford to increase his ability to get around the country more easily. This arrangement with the Roscommon County Council was heavily influenced by the fact that some of the best fly fishing in the country could be found in the lakes in the Roscommon area and close to Roscommon town. After two years, with little prospects of a surgical position in ophthalmology in Ireland and with the war beginning to show signs of ending, my father decided to reapply for a position in England by applying for a permit to the United Kingdom Permit office in Dublin which he received because he had been domiciled in the UK since 1925. He then opened discussions with the Camborne-Redruth Miners and General Hospital group in Redruth, Cornwall in May 1945 and subsequently applied for the post of Honorary Ophthalmic Surgeon there.

Waterford Hospital Services 1940s:

St. Patricks Hospital, Waterford was originally opened as a workhouse on 15th March 1841 costing in or around £10,000 and was designed to house 900 people, but during the great famine of 1848, was inundated by many more and eventually closed in 1920. Nursing care was provided by the Sisters of Mercy from 1883 to 1990. In 1921, St. Patrick's Hospital was designated as the City and County Hospital, and the centre for medicine, general surgery and orthopaedics as well as providing a casualty department for emergencies. Hospital services and the various medical specialties for the City and County of Waterford were well established and relatively good in the '50s but were spread widely throughout the city. Obstetrics and gynaecology services were provided at Airmount Hospital and were managed by the Medical Missionaries of Mary nuns. Psychiatry services were provided at St. Otteran's Hospital where a resident medical superintendent officer lived on site with his family. Ardkeen Chest Hospital, which was a sanatorium set up to treat TB patients, consisted of several large, isolated blocks of inpatient buildings furnished with open terraced verandas for maximum ventilation for the patients. Each unit was self-contained suitable for long-stay patients with chronic chest conditions. Part of one of these units had access to a surgical theatre to facilitate examinations under anaesthesia such as bronchoscopy and a radiology facility for a visiting chest surgeon and radiologist. As well as these state-run institutions, the County and City Infirmary, funded by a private trust, employed a general physician, general surgeon and a general practitioner experienced in maternity practice, which catered for citizens of Waterford who wish to be treated privately.

Chapter 3
Foundation of Ophthalmological Services in Waterford 1945

Ophthalmology services consisted of basic refraction testing for glasses and outpatient eye examinations but to my knowledge, were only carried out in ill-equipped general practitioner's dispensary clinics throughout the Waterford city and county area under the care of Dr. J.P Duggan. With his retirement in Jan. 1945, a temporary honorary post in ophthalmology for the County and City of Waterford, based at St. Patrick's Hospital and the County and City Infirmary, became available. In July of that year, my father was appointed to the post by Waterford City manager at the time, S.J. Moynihan. Finally, in December 1945, at a meeting of the Local Appointments Committee (LAC), my father was appointed as ophthalmic surgeon to Waterford City and County Hospital group which involved seeing outpatients in a large empty room on the ground floor of St. Patrick's Hospital in Waterford and in St. Joseph's Hospital in Dungarvan. However, due to local politics, his inclusion to the City and County Infirmary was unsuccessful. While these basic facilities available to him at the time, allowed my father to see and examine eye patients as outpatients, there was still no actual facility for admitting patients to hospital for special eye care or to carry out eye surgical procedures. Approaches were then made by my father to the county manager, Mr. Liam Raftice and the Public Assistance Board, for the use of a section of the building at St. Patrick's Hospital which was vacant at the time, to be set up with an outpatient clinic on the ground floor and a possible 12 bed inpatient unit with an eye operating theatre facility on the upper floor, the latter of which had been previously used to house greyhounds. St. Joseph Hospital in Dungarvan was to become an outpatient eye clinic for the West Waterford area.

In 1947, finances by the Waterford Board of Public Assistance were made available to make basic modifications to the building during which the empty room upstairs was partitioned off to provide an inpatient ward area and a small operating room, following which an application was made to the Minister for Health at the time, Dr. James Ryan. Almost a year later following a letter of approval from the Department of Health, for the establishment of an ophthalmic unit in the County Hospital as St. Patrick's in Waterford, a medical inspector was sent by the Department to inspect the building and his report to be subsequently sent to the board and to my father for their comments.

In the meantime, the hospital group in Redruth, Cornwall were requesting him to attend for an interview which they said would be necessary before any appointment could be made. However, his decision to remain in Ireland, and not to attend for interview in England, was greeted with great disappointment by the hospital group in the UK as evidenced by the number of letters received from the secretary superintendent in Redruth.

Tower Hill, Ferrybank and 128 The Quay 1947–1956:

Shortly after his LAC appointment, in August 1946, the family moved from Oakville in Clonmel to Tower Hill, Ferrybank, Waterford when I was just 10 years of age. Once my father had decided to cancel the UK arrangements and remain in Ireland to work, and because it would take some time to set up the facilities at Saint Patrick's hospital, my father purchased 128, The Quay and set up private practice rooms there.

"The Inspector Calls" – Dept. of Health Inspection:

Almost a year later, following a letter of approval from the Department of Health, for the establishment of an ophthalmic unit in the County Hospital at St. Patrick's in Waterford, a medical inspector was sent by the Department, to inspect the building, with his report subsequently sent to the board and to my father for their comments. The report, which was extremely detailed, covered all aspects of the building and the services to be required. It also included the outpatient's medical examination and patient waiting areas on the ground floor, as well as the already constructed operating theatre and the two six bed inpatient wards on the first floor. There were also references to facilities for in- patients and to the equipping of the operating theatre.

It was proposed to have the sterilizing done in the general hospital CSSD sterilizer initially. He also insisted that the unit must be completely separated from and have nothing to do or any communication with the General Hospital, which would also apply to the staff.

RAC Response:

In his reply, my father stated he was prepared to only use his own equipment for operating and to do all the dressings personally. He also informed them that he was prepared to start work in the unit with one qualified nurse with ophthalmic experience, but that she must have time off duty which would necessitate a second person, and that one nurse alone would not be sufficient. He also suggested that there be one or two nurse probationers in training and agreed that the unit and staff would have to be independent from the general hospital.

Final Decision:

In 1949, following a letter of approval in principle by the Department of Health to the Waterford Board of Public Assistance, the following letter was sent to my father from the secretary, Mr. Flanagan, which read as follows: "I enclose (a): A.29/73 dated 20th December, 1948 received from the Department of Health on 7th January, conveying the Minister's approval in principle to the establishment of an ophthalmic unit at the County Hospital, Waterford and (b): an extract from the report of the medical inspector who inspected the unit. I am directed by the manager to request you to submit a report in conjunction with the county surveyor as to the structural alterations necessary and to the equipment and staffing required in such a unit. I am further directed by the manager to inform you that in the meantime until the completion and operation of the new unit, the practice of performing major ophthalmic surgical operations in the general theatre and accommodating the patients in the general wards afterward, be discontinued as directed by the Department of Health".

Specialised Eye Healthcare Nursing Initiated:

Following an agreement to comply with the report on completion of the work and to send his report of work to be done to the building structure by the board, Sister Louis Ryan, a Presentation

Order religious nun, was allowed to attend Moorfields Eye Hospital, London on the Ophthalmic Nursing Diploma and Eye Theatre training courses, returning a year later to head up the specialised nursing eye care side of the unit.

1950–1959: First Surgical Eye Department – St. Patrick's Hospital, Waterford City and County:

Following minor structural alterations to the outpatient area on the ground floor and minimal changes to the surgical unit on the first floor, together with the purchase of surgical instruments suitable for the carrying out of cataract, glaucoma, squint procedures and eye emergencies, the unit was officially opened in 1950. As there was a large backlog of patients with surgically treatable conditions on the waiting list, my father lost no time in expediting the service and in providing an inpatient eye care service for eye emergencies for Waterford City and County which quickly extended into the surrounding areas. Previously, all patients requiring basic in-patient eye care, for all eye conditions, had no alternative but to go to Dublin to the Royal Victoria Eye and Ear Hospital, where there was a waiting list for admissions. An example of one who was treated by my father for an eye problem in the unit at St. Patricks hospital, without the need to go to Dublin, was, a

Waterford Public Assistance Bill for hospitalisation

Jacqueline Mathews from Grantstown, who received special eye care treatment for several weeks under the Waterford Board of Public Assistance during Nov. 1952, for which she received a bill for one pound, one shilling but was able to remain in Waterford while being treated.

Advances in Cataract Surgery – Intracapsular, the Next Step – 1950s:

The basic operation carried out at the time was the extracapsular operation which involved the use of the Graefe knife to open the eye. With the increasing volume of surgery, over a period, my father accumulated many new surgical skills as his experience and knowledge expanded. This was stimulated mostly by his many visits to the major well-known eye centres throughout Europe where he learned new surgical techniques for the various more complicated eye conditions. One of these clinics was the well-known Barraquer clinic in Barcelona, Spain, which had a special viewing chamber for surgeons to observe some of the best surgeons in the world operate. One example of these demonstrated skills on offer, involved the safe transition from the outdated extracapsular cataract technique at the time to the more modern intracapsular one. With the development of an enzyme called Alpha-Chymotrypsin to loosen the zonular fibres holding the cataract in place, a safer removal of the whole lens could be achieved with a suction cup instrument called the Erysiphake to physically grasp the lens for easy removal from the eye. This technique was subsequently improved on using a frozen probe tip, a technique called cryoextraction. To the best of my knowledge, my father was one of the first persons in Ireland to convert from the older extracapsular to the more advanced Barraquer intracapsular technique but continued to use the Graefe knife to make an ab interno incision.

Chapter 4
Replacement of the Cataract with an Artificial Lens Implant:

Because cataracts are hazy opacities that grow inside the natural focusing lens of the eye, the removal of a cataract naturally leaves the eye without the capacity to focus light through to the back of the eye, so that everything appears hazy and blurry to the patient necessitating the wearing of very heavy thick spectacle lenses to see clearly. The thought of implanting a man-made artificial lens into the eye after removal of the cataract, had been in Dr. Harold Ridley's mind for some time. Following a comment made by a medical student, Steve Parry while watching him operate at St. Thomas' Hospital, London, as to why a focusing lens was not being used to replace the cataract, Ridley decided that the time had come to design an artificial lens that would fit inside the eye

Harold Ridley (1906–2001):

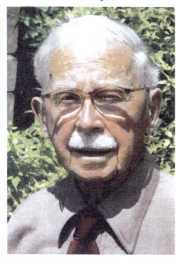

Harold Ridley

Nicholas Harold Lloyd Ridley, FRCS (Eng.), Fellow of Royal Society (FRS), was born in 1906 at Kibworth, Leicester, UK. His father, Nicholas Charles Ridley, FRCS, was a consultant ophthalmic surgeon at the Leicester Royal Infirmary. After a basic schooling in Godalming, Surrey, young Nicholas Ridley attended Pembroke College in Cambridge University, from 1924 until he commenced the study of medicine at St. Thomas' Hospital,

London in 1927, where he completed his basic medical training in 1930. This was followed by a two-year period working as a junior hospital doctor in the ophthalmic department at St. Thomas' Hospital under consultant Mr. A. Cyril Hudson, attaining his FRCS qualification in 1932 at 25 years of age. While at St. Thomas' hospital, consultant Geoffrey Doyne, who was also a consultant at Moorfields Eye Hospital, advised him to undergo training at Moorfields which he subsequently undertook for a two-year period working with the most prestigious of world-class eye surgeons. Following a year as a ship surgeon and a period of residency at Moorfields Eye Hospital, Ridley carried out a visit to the Viennese School of Ophthalmology, and to eye hospitals in Budapest and Munich in 1935.

Having studied a great deal on cataract surgical techniques by such a variety of surgeons, he became convinced that the extracapsular technique of removing the cataract and leaving the capsule behind was the best procedure and was eventually the one he adopted later when it came to lens implantation. In 1938, he was made a permanent consultant at Moorfields Eye Hospital and became involved in restructuring the education and training of junior eye doctors at the hospital.

In 1941, Ridley was appointed temporary major, in the Royal Army Medical Corps, following which, he was sent by Sir Stewarts Duke- Elder, then a high-ranking ophthalmic officer in the British Army, to Ghana, the Gold Coast of West Africa, where he was appointed part-time sanitary officer at headquarters in the capital city of Accra. Together with Brigadier, G.M. Findlay, A. M. S., he pursued investigations on blinding eye conditions caused by Onchocerciasis (River Blindness), vitamin A deficiency and leprosy, which were endemic in the area at the time. These efforts in tropical ophthalmology led to his early involvement with the Royal Commonwealth Society for the Blind lead by Sir John Wilson. The society was a major consortium of government and non-governmental organisations dedicated to fighting blindness especially in the developing world.

Following his discharge as a Major from the army in 1945, he returned to the UK with a mandate from the government to supervise vitamin A deficiency for those in institutional care.

In 1946, Ridley opened a private consulting room at 53, Harley St., London, where he lived and practised for the following 40 years. He served as a post-war consultant ophthalmologist to the Ministry of Defence until 1971 and, from 1965 to 1971, was a member of the Expert Advisory panel on Parasitic Diseases for the World Health Organisation.

RAF Canopy Windscreen Eye Injuries:

Some of the injuries were sustained by RAF pilots during the Battle of Britain, in air combat and dogfights with the Luftwaffe, were the serious face and eye injuries from the implosion of the cockpit windscreen canopies which provided little protection from enemy gunfire. Whereas many of them lost some if not all their sight from these injuries, several of them retained pieces of the windscreen in their eyes including Squadron leader Gordon Mouse Cleaver of 601 Squadron, who had retained splinters of windscreen remaining in his eye.

While seeing a number of these retired wounded pilots, Ridley noticed that whereas retained pieces of metal inside the eye gradually corrode leading to complete loss of vision and a blind eye, retained Perspex from these injuries remain totally inert.

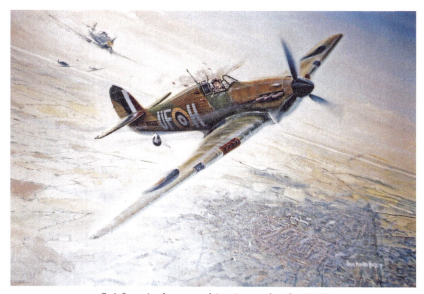

Spitfire airplane used in air combat by RAF

Rayners and the First Intraocular lens Implant:

With this in mind, he contacted John Pike, the optical scientist at Rayners of London, who had recently been working on Ridley's electric ophthalmoscope. Within months, they had worked out a design for an artificial lens to fit inside the eye at surgery after removal of the cataract. Because of its suitability within the eye and its weight in water compared to glass, the material chosen for the implant was poly methyl methacrylate (PMMA) or Perspex made by ICI in the UK. As plastic material could not be autoclaved at high temperatures for sterilisation purposes, a chemical method of sterilisation using Cetrimide was decided on. On the 29th November 1949, Harold Ridley carried out his first intraocular lens implant operation on a cataract patient at St. Thomas' Hospital, London assisted only by his theatre nurse, Doreen Ogg, in total secrecy. Whereas the procedure went extremely well, the patient ended up extremely short sighted with a refraction of -14 D but with extremely good vision. The following week, he performed a similar operation at Moorfields Eye Hospital with similar results which necessitated changing the power of the implant subsequently. With the help of John Pike from Rayners, the optical results improved, but without any major physical support within the eye, the implant tended to dislocate requiring its removal, which was extremely disheartening for Ridley especially when the patient had experienced good vision post operatively.

UK Controversy Oxford Congress July 1951:

For a year after his first operation, Ridley, being extremely aware of criticism from his colleagues at Moorfields and St. Thomas' hospitals, conducted his first series of intraocular lens implantations secretly at St. Thomas' Hospital. Unknown to himself, a patient of his unwittingly attended Mr. Frederick Ridley (no relation) at Moorfields Hospital with a problem, who in turn alerted Sir Stewart Duke -Elder to these procedures. At the UK Congress of ophthalmology at Oxford in July 1951, Harold Ridley presented his results bringing with him two patients with good outcomes for the doctors to examine. Following his presentation, a caucus of ophthalmologists ridiculed his results, one of which was Sir Stewart Duke-Elder, who refused to even examine Ridley's patients who had attended especially for the meeting. In the following year, at the American Academy of Ophthalmology and

Otolaryngology, Dr. Derek Vail, editor of the American Journal of Ophthalmology, adopted a similar attitude being extremely dismissive of Ridley's results.

Intraocular Lens Implant Waterford:

Being familiar with Mr. Harold Ridley's presentation of his series of the first intraocular lens implants at the Oxford Congress in 1951, and with Mr. Peter Choyce, a well-known surgeon also in the UK, who was working with Rayner at the time developing his anterior chamber intraocular lens implant, my father was aware of the scenario that was about to develop regarding the potential of lens implantation. At the time, he had a 54-year-old Waterford patient, Mr. Larry Guinan, who had a successful cataract procedure done by him, but who was having extreme difficulty at work and driving with the standard very thick spectacles glasses he was forced to wear to see clearly at his job after the operation. Following detailed consultation with Rayner, a Choyce anterior chamber intraocular lens implant was manufactured to Mr. Guinan's eye specifications and was inserted in a separate operation by my father. To my knowledge, this was one of the first intraocular lens implant procedure to be carried out in Ireland at the

---

Waterford Man Can See Again

A 54-YEAR-OLD Waterford man who had lost vision in both eyes had his sight restored as the result of a unique operation involving the replacement of the natural lenses with acrytic plastic lense.

He is Mr. Larry Guinan, Ard-na-Greine, who, due to the skill of on eminent Waterford surgeon oculist, can now read and go to the pictures again.

Mr. Guinan had worked on the docks for 25 years. Then his sight began to fail and gradually his vision became so restricted that, he said, "I could see only shadows".

CATARACTS REMOVED

In the Eye Unit of St. Patrick's Hospital Waterford, the cataracts were removed and he got the usual thick glasses. But he could not get on with those glasses. In a further operation, plastic lenses were put into the centre of each eye. The second operation was successful. Mr. Guinan was examined at a meeting of eye surgeons from all over the world.

A series of somewhat similar operations was carried out in the hospital in 1957 and 1958 but this is believed to be the first time, however, the operation was done in Ireland entailing the insertion of plastic lenses inside both eyes.

time, which the local Waterford press lost no time in reporting. Subsequently, Mr. Guinan had his other eye operated successfully. This was followed by several further lens implantations over the course of the next few years.

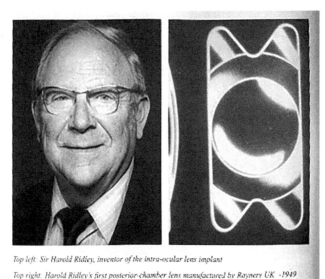

Top left: Sir Harold Ridley, inventor of the intra-ocular lens implant
Top right: Harold Ridley's first posterior-chamber lens manufactured by Rayners UK -1949

Intraocular Lens Implant in Ireland – Newspaper Report

Celebrating 50 Years of the IOL

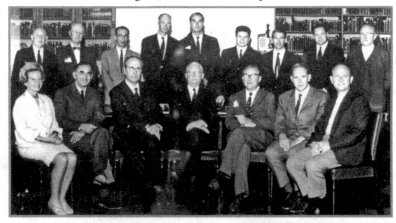

IIIC Founders at the Inaugural Meeting 14 July 1966 in London, England
Pictured are: John Pike (Rayner), Robert Murto (guest), Michael Roper-Hall (UK), Slava Fyodorov (USSR), Neil Dallas (UK), Sandy Brown (UK), Alexander Rubenstein (UK), Warren Reese (USA), Leonard Lurie (UK), Jorn Boberg-Ans and Sonja Boberg-Ans (Denmark), Cees Binkhorst (The Netherlands), D. Peter Choyce (UK), Harold Ridley (UK), Benedetto Strampelli (Italy), Edward Epstein (South Africa)

International Intraocular Implant Council Foundation (IIIC), 1966

International Intraocular Lens Implant Council (IIIC):

With the continuing controversy raging on for 10 years, Harold Ridley convened a small club of international cataract and implant surgeons in London in 1966, called the International Intraocular Implant Club, subsequently extending it to a council in which surgeons involved in lens implant surgery could convene internationally.

MCh National University of Ireland UCD and UK Faculty of Ophthalmology:

Shortly after being appointed to the post of ophthalmic surgeon in Waterford, he started his study preparation for the master's degree in surgery examination at UCD. One of the textbooks he used, and which helped him greatly to be subsequently conferred with the MCh degree, was Vogt's Atlas on Slit Lamp Microscopy of the Eye which had just been published.

Since leaving the UK, my father remained a member of the UK Faulty of Ophthalmology and was particularly friendly with D. Hudson of St. Thomas' Hospital in London. On one of his visits with the UK Faculty y to Rome, my father was presented with a medal from the Pope in May 1949 in recognition of his work. This

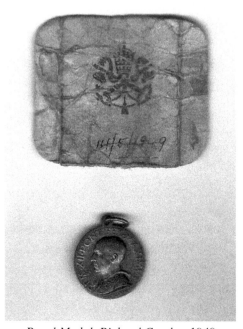

Papal Medal, Richard Condon,1949

stimulated him and his colleagues in Ireland to set up the Irish Faculty of Ophthalmology in the mid '50s, of which he became President subsequently.

Waterford Clinical Society:

With a long history of medical meetings for GP's and consultants in the Waterford area, the WCS was an extremely social group which met every month during the year and had an annual dinner around the Christmas or New Year period. The society provided a great communication between the different specialties and general practitioners which was of great benefit to the patients. My father, who was a great advocate of the society, was made President and wore the chain of office during the '50s when the society was extremely active.

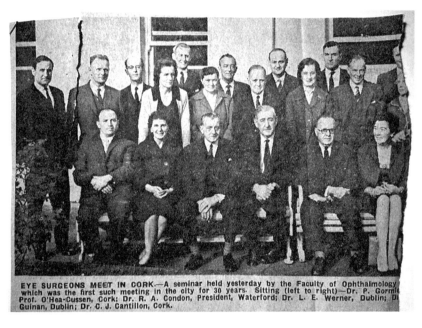

President Irish Faculty of Ophthalmology 1949

Industrialisation of Waterford – Increased Emergencies:

Starting in 1936, Waterford was one of the first cities in Ireland to manufacturer range cookers and stoves for domestic heating, culminating in the Waterford Stanley heavy engineering company at Bilberry. This was followed in the early '40s, with the arrival of Waterford Crystal in Kilcohan and its rapid expansion into

Johnstown from where it eventually took off before finally establishing itself on the Cork Road development site. Whereas the safety measures taken by many of these companies were incorporated into the industrial work practices by NISO and the larger companies, there was a major increase in eye accidents attending for eye casualty treatments.

With the continued attraction of Waterford as an area for development, many construction companies became involved in the provision of accommodation for workers and factory buildings. Also, bearing in mind that laminated windscreens and car seatbelt legislation had not yet been introduced together with lax drink-driving laws, the numbers of road traffic accidents involving eye injuries attending the clinic started to escalate. Whereas my father, as a single part-time consultant, was responsible for the unit and its casualty department, he was fortunate during annual leave and attendance in court, to be able to deputise some of the work to his colleague, Dr. Louis Ryan, who worked privately in Parnell St. and in Kilkenny.

1960–1976: Second Surgical Eye Department – Ardkeen Hospital Waterford City and County:

In 1957 the Minister for Health, Dr. James Ryan, proposed that Ardkeen Chest Hospital be converted to the proposed county hospital and in 1959, St Patrick's County Hospital services were transferred to Ardkeen Hospital with retention of St Patrick's as an elderly care centre. On the 1st of July 1960, the new Waterford Health Authority management was installed at Ardkeen Hospital. Whereas there were major improvements for general surgery, orthopaedics and general medicine, in that each one acquired additional ward and theatre space in separate sanatoria unit blocks, ophthalmology and ear nose and throat surgical and inpatient services were forced to share a single sanatorium unit block with no space for outpatients. In the case of ophthalmology, this had the result that the room used for eye theatre surgical work was the only space available in which to treat outpatients for the Waterford city area. This meant that to carry out routine surgical lists and emergency procedures, the room used for surgery had to be cleaned and disinfected to a standard suitable for intraocular eye operations, which was not an entirely safe situation.

Unfortunately, with no other option, the practice of eye surgery in Ardkeen was forced to continue with this compromise. With a stable population of 100,000 for the city and county of Waterford, the unit was found capable of managing the routine surgical demands of the population at the time. In 1970, my father Richard Augustine Condon became ill with lung cancer, coming under the care of Mr. Desmond Kneafsey, visiting chest surgeon from Galway University Hospital. After a relatively short period of hospitalisation in Ardkeen Hospital, he died in February 1974.

Chapter 5
Basic Education and University Medical Training

My Early Education:

Following my secondary school education at De La Salle College in Waterford and Clongowes Wood College, in 1955, I applied to University College Cork for admission to the pre-medicine programme year and qualified with a MB, BCh, BAO from the National University of Ireland (NUI) in 1960. Two 6-month periods were then spent as an internship in St. Vincent's Hospital, Dublin and St. Michael's Hospital, Dun Laoghaire before leaving for the UK.

United Kingdom 1961:

With very little prospect of a post graduate career in medicine or surgery in Ireland at the time, most Irish graduates were encouraged to look to the UK or the USA for further development of their careers. Based on my father's UK background, I immediately set my sights on London and started looking for a hospital house officer post in the London area. However, without a London address, I had little hope of entering the London scenario. In my enquiries, I was extremely fortunate to learn that a Dr. Tom Cleary from Clonmel who was in the same year as me and who had qualified in Cork in UCC, was working as a junior house officer in the Hospital of St. John and St. Elizabeth, in St. Johns Wood, North London. With an introduction by Tom to the hospital manager, I received an offere to take on short term locum work at the hospital, and being unemployed, was available to start work quickly, but only for short periods at a time. As I needed to get more experience in medicine and surgery at senior house officer level, and as some of the top consultants in London worked out of

St. John and St. Elizabeth Hospital, I decided to wait for the next posts to be advertised. In the meantime, I rented out a bedsitter in the St. John's Wood and Swiss Cottage area and applied for locum relief work at various NHS hospitals throughout the London area.

During that period, I got incredible experience of working in a great variety of different hospitals and casualty departments and was eventually appointed senior house officer in medicine and surgery for a year at St. John and St. Elizabeth hospital, subsequently benefiting greatly from working there.

Ophthalmological Career – An Introduction 1962:

During the nine months spent as senior house officer in medicine and surgery at St. John and St. Elizabeth where I was exposed to a great variety of medicine and surgery, I was becoming extremely interested in taking up medicine as a career. On returning home during holiday periods, my father who was 66 years of age at the time, suggested to me as to whether I might consider a career in ophthalmology with a possibility of taking over his practice eventually. As a result, I decided to apply for a senior house officer post in the Croydon Eye Unit at Mayday Hospital in Surrey, UK to work under the supervision of Mr. Dermot Pierse, Mr. Ray Davies, and Mr. Patrick Holmes Sellors for a six-month period.

Within a week of my application, I was accepted for the post and started work a week before Christmas 1962. Mayday Hospital, which was a general hospital in the centre of Croydon, had an extremely active eye department with a helpful registrar from New Zealand, Dr. Hilton Le Grice, who guided me technically in my first job in ophthalmology. Mr. Pierse's secretary, Mrs. Sheila Tant and the office staff were also extremely supportive in arranging my accommodation. Being terribly conscious of my total lack of knowledge in ophthalmology, and as a beginner in the specialty, I stuck as closely as I could in the clinics and operating room to Hilton and the staff who provided technical guidance as I made my way along for the first few months. As a result, I had very little direct contact with the consultants as my ophthalmic education continued. It did not take too long to figure out that I was going to be happy in ophthalmology and decided there and then to sign up for the primary Fellowship of the Royal College of Surgeons (FRCS) basic science course in the Nuffield Institute at the Royal

College of Surgeons, Lincoln's Inn Fields, central London, which was due to start in September later that year. As both the course and the accommodation at the Nuffield, was quite expensive, I decided that for the 3-month period from July to September, to apply for general practice locum work and ended up working in two separate practices in the north of the country, and another in Bedford.

While the day-to-day work tended to be quite mundane, the house visits to patients allowed me to see the countryside outside the London area and was far less claustrophobic than hospital practice. Nor was it short of excitement in that on one occasion, I was called on a Sunday afternoon to see a patient who had collapsed with status asthmaticus, and who was unconscious and totally cyanotic on arrival at the house. Following an injection of aminophylline and some ephedrine combined with mouth-to-mouth respiration and intermittent cardiac resuscitation, I managed to bring her around and save her life. I subsequently heard from the GP, that following a similar attack, she eventually died.

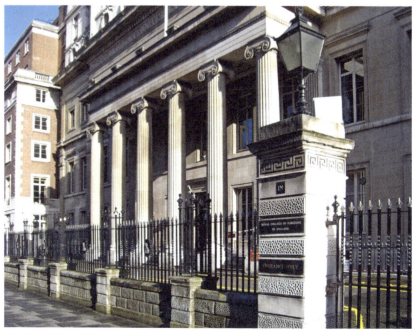

Nuffield College of Basic Surgical Sciences, RCS, London

Primary Fellowship of the Royal College of Surgeons in England Basic Science Course:

For all doctors who wish to become surgeons in any specialty, the primary fellowship examination in surgery, or Primary FRCS, must be passed before the final specialty exam can be taken. This examination which involves applied anatomy, physiology, biochemistry, pharmacology, and others, is designed to lay the foundations in the basic sciences, in preparation for the second part of the exam. The FRCS part 2, is more specifically surgically orientated, concentrating on the various specialties such as general, neuro, cardiothoracic, genitourinary, vascular, plastic surgery, ear nose and throat and ophthalmology. Because the wealth of information is so vast, and the examinations involve written and oral tests, it is necessary to take time off from a busy hospital practice to find time to study and eventually to proceed to the second part. It was while living in accommodation at the Nuffield Institute of Basic Sciences having dinner, when we received the tragic news of the assassination of the President of the United States, John F. Kennedy. No one will ever forget that evening of November 1963 and it remained the subject of conversation for a long time thereafter.

Participants for the course were extremely varied coming from all parts of the globe but more especially from Australia, many of whom would eventually progress to general surgery for the second part. From the ophthalmic point of view, there were three of us which included a well-known Irish ophthalmologist, Tom Casey from Limerick who was already a consultant at the Queen Victoria Cornea-Plastic and Eye Bank Unit in East Grinstead, Frank Lavery from Dublin and me. As to the course itself, Prof. Last, Prof of Applied Anatomy and Prof. Barry Wyke, Professor of physiology and pharmacology, were top quality speakers and lecturers which made it easier to absorb the knowledge and update us since our earlier days in first and second medicine years.

At the end of the three-month period of hard studying, the Irish Primary Fellowship examination took place in January 1964 at the College in St Stephen's Green, Dublin. Whereas the written papers were not too difficult, the oral examination for me as a prospective ophthalmologist, involved the most complex respiratory pulmonary function tests in physiology and the musculature of the sole of the foot in anatomy, which for one hoping to practice ophthalmology, seemed totally superfluous. With the Primary FRCS achieved, Frank Lavery from Dublin and I went on a skiing holiday to Ehrwald in Austria for two weeks, after which I immediately applied for a senior house officer post at the Royal Eye/St. Thomas' Hospital training programme in ophthalmology in south London, while Frank applied for a post in the Croydon Eye Unit.

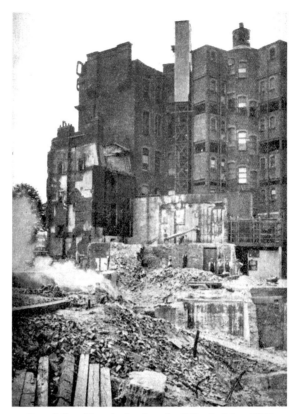

Royal Eye Hospital, after the Blitz in May, 1941

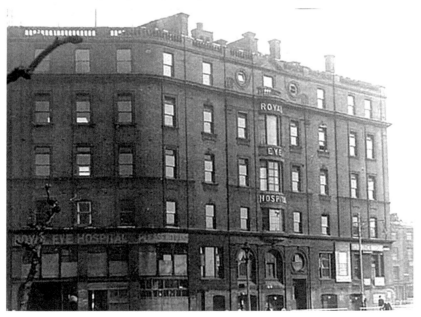

Royal Eye Hospital following reconstruction

Chapter 6
Becoming an Ophthalmologist – 1960's

Royal Eye /St. Thomas'/Lambeth Hospital South London Rotation Group Programme: 1963–1967

Royal Eye Hospital:

Because of their situation directly across the river from the Houses of Parliament in the Lambeth area, both St. Thomas' and the Royal Eye Hospitals were badly damaged in 1941 by the bombings during the Blitz. When the war ended, due to their major significance in the provision of essential services, both hospitals were quickly rebuilt and restored in the 1950s to fully working status and as teaching hospital for training. After its incorporation into the NHS in 1948, the Royal Eye continued as the major eye

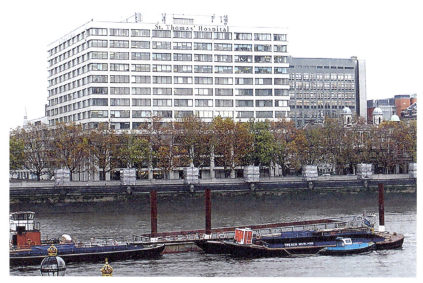

St. Thomas' Hospital rebuilt after the war

hospital in southeast London until 1974, when its services and as a training centre for ophthalmology were relocated to St. Thomas' Hospital. Within a short while afterwards, the hospital became derelict and was eventually demolished leaving a site on which the current McLaren House residency for students at London South Bank University stands.

Following a successful interview, I started as a senior house officer at the Royal Eye Hospital, St. Georges Circus, South London in 1964. The facilities at the hospital included several eye operating theatres, inpatient beds, outpatient clinics, a busy casualty department, a laboratory staffed by technicians, and a small radiology department. The hospital was managed by a very competent hospital administrator, a Ms Barber and her staff. The consultant staff included doctors Alistair Cameron, Ronald Pitts-Crick, Peter Clover, Doreen Birks, Alan Friedman, Ms Dollar, Ms Savoury and Professor Arnold Sorsby.

Professor Arnold Sorsby, CBE, became Dean of the medical school from 1934 to 38 and from 1934 to 1966, was Research Professor of Ophthalmology at the Royal College of Surgeons and the Royal Eye. In his role as research Professor at the College and the Royal Eye, his research into the causes of blindness and genetic diseases were legendary. He was awarded the Sir Arthur Keith medal for services to the College in 1966. This was followed by his appointment as Commander of the Order of the British Empire (CBE) in respect of his national and international service to ophthalmology and for his work with the WHO advisory panel on Trachoma and the International Association for the Prevention of Blindness. I also had the opportunity to work with Arnold Sorsby and publish a chapter on "Maternal Disorder" in his volumes of Modern Ophthalmology Vol. 2:1972 published by Butterworths of London. Following an extremely scientific illustrious career, he retired in 1966 and continued to work on committees until his death in 1980.

Cataract Extraction Technique – Extracapsular to Intracapsular:

At the time, the standard cataract operation carried out by some of the older consultants was the extracapsular technique ab interno approach using the Graefe knife to make the incision.

However, most of the more recently trained consultants were using the intracapsular techniques like that of my father. Apart from the cataract procedure, most of the consultants also had developed special interests in varied aspects of ophthalmology. For instance, Dr. Ronald Pitts- Crick, a specialist in squint and glaucoma surgery, who had been developing a surgical microscope with Keeler Ophthalmics since 1956, had his original prototype microscope based at the Royal Eye Hospital operating theatre for the resident doctors to use in their training.

A more advanced prototype was subsequently demonstrated at the Oxford Congress in 1958 and the 18th International Congress in Brussels. Alan Friedmann was also working with Keeler Ophthalmics in the development of the Friedmann Visual Field Analyser screening instrument for the early diagnosis of glaucoma and neurological diseases affecting the visual pathways. There was also considerable interest by all the consultants in the use of the Zeiss "Jumbo" Light Coagulator for the treatment of diabetic retinopathy and retinal vascular diseases. Ms Doreen Birks specialised in corneal transplantation and corneal diseases.

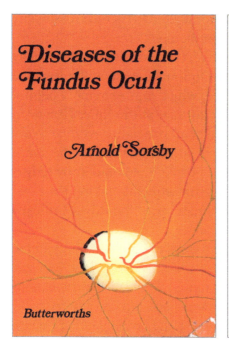

Arnold Sorsby book on Retinal Diseases

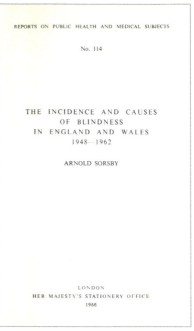

Arnold Sorsby. Blindness in UK, Report, 1948–62

Diploma in Ophthalmology (Edin.):

As a senior house officer, I was provided with accommodation and lived in the hospital being on call at night for casualty and working with the consultants during the day at their outpatient clinics at the Royal Eye, assisting at operating lists and was responsible for the medical care of the inpatients. During the working day, being a relative beginner at the job and not knowing too much about ophthalmology at the time, I was assisted by the registrar, Dr. Joseph Walsh, a Kerry man and supervised by the senior registrar who happened to be Dr. John Blake from Cork. Dr. Blake had just finished his training at the Royal Eye and was preparing to return to Dublin to take up an assistant consultant post at the Royal Victoria Eye and Ear Hospital there.

My immediate colleagues were Dr. John Griffiths from Wales, and Dr. James McGrand from Northern Ireland, who were excellent at sharing information and participating in discussions on the various patients we had seen during the day and provided good company when we were not working. Whereas the practical experience of dealing with patients with eye problems was quite different to dealing with those without ophthalmic problems, it did not take long for me as a junior doctor to become reasonably competent at dealing with their problems.

During my year at the Royal Eye, I was able to use the holiday period to attend the Moorfields Diploma course at the Institute of Ophthalmology in Judd Street, which was extremely helpful in consolidating my knowledge to date at the time. However, even though the consultants and senior registrar were actively involved in teaching sessions, there still was a need for the junior eye doctor to increase his or her basic academic knowledge, especially if one was considering subsequently taking the Final Fellowship ophthalmology examinations of the Royal Colleges of Surgeons.

The shortage of the major textbooks in ophthalmology in the small library at the hospital which mostly included the journals of the day, made it necessary for those taking subsequent examinations to acquire their own textbooks and reading materials. In this respect, my registrar colleagues at the hospital either bought their textbooks privately or rented them from Lewis Library in Gower St. returning them on passing their exams.

In my case I decided to use my off-duty time, in the Senate library of the University of London, in Malet Street off Russell Square. At that time, medical and postgraduate university students had free access and the library was open in the evenings and on Saturdays, when I was not on duty at the hospital. Having been well used to the intense study required in preparation for the Primary Fellowship examination, it was a great pleasure to be able to sit down undisturbed and study the diseases of the eye which was totally relevant to my hospital practice. The availability of the 12 volumes of Duke Elder's System of Ophthalmology and the facilities at the library, offered a complete change to the constant demands of active hospital life.

Not having any friends outside the hospital, at weekends when not on duty, I often walked around Westminster, attending mass at the Abbey, and exploring the area north of the Thames. It was about this time while being on duty on 24th January 1964, that Sir Winston Churchill died. It was fascinating to watch his funeral procession passing by the Royal Eye Hospital on its way to Westminster from my room overlooking the cavalcade.

During my year as a SHO at the Roya Eye Hospital, and ready to move on to the second-year spell at Lambeth, I was glad to have found the opportunity to go to Edinburgh to take the DO exam witch I subsequently passed.

Lambeth Hospital, Brook Drive, London, SE11 1965–1966:

This second year as senior house officer in the Royal Eye Hospital rotation programme involved working and living at the Lambeth Hospital where I was provided with accommodation and subsistence. The Brook Drive area of Lambeth is well known as the birthplace of Charlie Chaplin who was born on 11th April 1889, in or around the time when the Lambeth hospital was founded. In later years, it had become part of the Royal Eye, St. Thomas' Hospital group, and was used as a support hospital. The unit at the Lambeth hospital on the third floor of Block C comprised a male and female ward with an eye operating theatre, and an anaesthetic and recovery area for patients undergoing ophthalmic surgical procedures. The unit was staffed by nurses from the St. Thomas' hospital group which included ward sister Greta Condon (no relation) originally from

Ferrybank, Waterford, theatre sister Thorogood and staff nurse Murphy. Surgical procedures for cataract, glaucoma, squint correction, and retinal detachment repair, were carried by Mr. Noel Moores, Mr. Alan Friedman, and the Royal Eye Hospital registrar and senior registrar in ophthalmology as part of their training. The consultants, senior registrar, and registrar who carried out surgery here, were also responsible for the SHO's surgical training as part of the group.

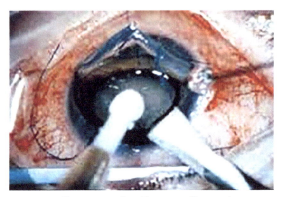

Extracapsular Cataract Extraction

As regards cataract surgery techniques, I began to see a marked change in that most of the consultants, including the registrar and senior registrar, preferred to use the ab externo intracapsular technique. This involved making a 12 mm sized incision from the outside of the eye in the 12 o'clock position with blade and scissors, injecting Alpha- Chymotrypsin around the edge of the cataract to dissolve the suspensory ligament of the lens, fixating the lens with a cryoprobe and extracting it from the eye. The incision was then sutured up with 5-0 black silk.

Gradually I became familiar with many surgical procedures such as the correction of squints in children and how to reattach the muscle correctly to the sclera. As time progressed, I became increasingly familiar with the consultants and thereby gained their confidence to be allowed to suture incisions and having access to the extremely delicate instruments they were using. I also became confident using magnification doing these procedures which at the time involved the BinoMag loupes which most of the consultants used around their heads while performing surgery. Gradually, I developed a completely new insight into the scope of ophthalmology and its close association to general medicine and the rest of the body.

Future Examinations 1966-1967:

With almost two years in ophthalmology behind me, it was time to start thinking about the basic examinations in the various subjects with a view to acquiring some ophthalmic qualifications, the first of which was the Diploma in Ophthalmology (DO), which I had already passed. However, ahead of me, was the challenge to acquire a Fellowship from one of the Royal Colleges that would be of great value in applying for future posts.

I finally decided to sit the Edinburgh exam and made enquiries into the syllabus, examination procedures and differences in emphasis that one College might have over the other. It transpired that Prof. Barry Cullen, a Dublin graduate, was the consultant neuro ophthalmologist attached to the college and regarded as a world authority with a strong influence of neurology on the examination. I immediately hired out from Lewis's library in Gower Street, both of David Cogan's books and Frank Walsh's Atlas on neuro ophthalmology, which I started to devour. As the examination also involved the candidate having to make a full neurological examination of an actual patient with various neurological conditions, it seemed difficult at the time as to how while working purely in ophthalmology and at a distance from general medicine, that this could be achieved.

To overcome this deficiency, I took the liberty of contacting the senior registrar in neurology at the West End Hospital for Nervous Diseases in Dean Street, central London which was attached to Queen Square Hospital for Nervous Diseases, for permission to attend ward rounds in an observer capacity. With a full scheduled commitment during the day at the Royal Eye, an arrangement was made with the neurology senior registrar and the consultant in charge of the patients, that would allow me to attend in the evening time when the registrar was making his rounds admitting patients, so that I might become familiar with the finer points in the examination and diagnosis of patients with these conditions and their current management. With further enquiries, I also discovered that demyelinating diseases such as multiple sclerosis were, for some unknown reason, extremely prevalent in Scotland. As my duties as a SHO in having to carry out a full physical examination of patients admitted for eye surgery, I became extremely adept at including a full neurological assessment in my examination of patients for their eye operations.

Royal Eye Hospital, Surbiton, Surrey:

Following the damage to the hospital at South Park in May 1941, a large residential property at Upper Brighton Rd. in Surbiton, Surrey was purchased to accommodate the patients until December 1944, during which period the Southwark building had been restored. However, with the appointment of Mr. Timothy Tyrell and Mr. Peter Clover, the hospital continued to provide an ophthalmology service to the borough of Kingston and the surrounding area. It also continued to provide an extension to the Royal Eye rotation training programme at SHO and Registrar level which is how I ended up as a SHO for 3 months there, following my nine months at the Lambeth. Accommodation for the resident medical staff on duty was available in the gate lodge on the property and was extremely quiet and private. Being far from the bustle of central London, it was a most peaceful place to find time to catch up with my studies. With limited casualty exposure and limited theatre and outpatient duties, it was a great opportunity to prepare for the Fellowship exam.

Eric John Arnott, FRCS, DOMS (1929–2011):

At Surbiton, I assisted Mr. Eric Arnott who had been appointed as a third consultant to the hospital in addition to the Royal Eye Hospital group with facilities for surgical procedure at Surbiton. He had also just been appointed as a consultant to the Charing Cross Hospital group which was undergoing major reorganisation at the time with plans to build a new hospital at Fulham in early 1971. For cataracts, he was doing a straightforward intracapsular operation using a 12-millimetre incision with an ab externo blade and scissors but could also do an ab interno incision using a Graefe knife and closing the incision with a 5-0 black silk mattress suture. In the management of retinal detachment cases, I was with him when we carried out some of the earlier scleral buckling procedures for retinal detachment repair but using newer type soft silastic sponge material to indent the sclera over the retinal tear area.

Being from the well-known Arnott family of Arnott's prestigious store in Dublin and educated at Trinity College Dublin, I got on very well with him, to the extent that he invited me to use the indoor pool at the RAC Club in Central London. At the time, he was partial owner of the Phoenix Park Racecourse in Dublin with his brother John, which he seemed to visit quite often. In Ireland the name Arnott is synonymous with the well-established department store in Dublin with no relation to ophthalmology. It appears that Eric's great grandfather, John Arnott, first emigrated to Cork in 1837 from Fife, near Dundee, Scotland at the age of 23, in the hope of setting up a business which at first was unsuccessful. Moving to Belfast where he initially started a drapery business which was extremely successful, he returned to Cork to open his own drapery store there. Arnott's record as a retail entrepreneur made him an attractive business partner for William Cannock and Andrew Reid, who founded Arnott's in Dublin in 1843.

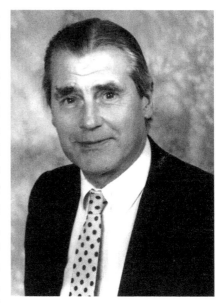

Mr. Eric Arnott, Consultant Royal Eye Hospital, 1960s 300

The Croydon Eye Unit, Mayday Hospital, Croydon, Surrey: 1966–1967

My first job as a registrar in ophthalmology was at the Croydon eye unit as part of the Royal Eye / St. Thomas group rotation program and began in May 1966. The building which was separate from the general hospital on Mayday Road, housed the eye outpatients and management secretarial sections and staff. All surgical procedures were carried out at Croydon General Hospital where theatre facilities for eye surgery and anaesthetics were available, as well as several beds reserved for eye in-patients. The consultants consisted of senior ophthalmologist, Mr. Ray Davies, (General ophthalmologist), Mr. Dermot Pierse (Anterior segment surgeon), Mr. Patrick Holmes Sellors (Retinal surgeon) and part timer, Mr. Hugh O'Donoghue (Lid, Lacrimal and Squint surgeon). The unit staff also included Ms Maeve-Ann Sandiford (Orthoptist), Dr. Jonathan Kersley, Contact Lens consultant and a local optometrist, Mr. Christopher Kerr who were all part of the unit. Dermot Pierse also had operating sessions at St. Anthony's Private Hospital which was run by The Daughters of the Cross in Cheam. Patrick Holmes Sellors also worked at St. Georges Hospital in Tooting. While working in this unit for several months previously as a total beginner in my basic introduction to ophthalmology in 1963, and under relatively close supervision by the registrar, I really had very little personal contact with any of the consultants. With 2 years' experience at SHO level and minor surgical experience, I was now in a much different position as I began my term as registrar and a lot more equipped to take on the challenging surgical aspects of the specialty than before. Realising the fact that as a registrar in the department, I would be working more closely with the consultants and secretaries in the organisation of things, I was a little apprehensive and somewhat intimidated during my first few weeks at work in May 1966.

During my first six months working as a registrar with the various consultants, I gradually gained experience at outpatient

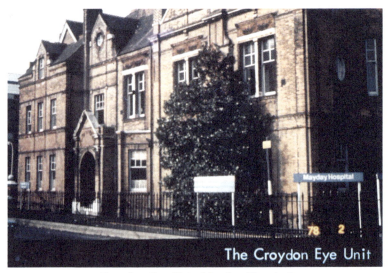

Croydon Eye Unit, Mayday Hospital

clinics and at presenting interesting cases to the department staff at monthly intervals. During this period, I observed the precise and sophisticated surgical techniques exhibited by Dermot Pierse in his cataract and corneal transplant cases. The standard cataract procedure was the intracapsular technique using a 12 mm corneo-scleral incision with a razor blade fragment and scissors followed by cryoextraction of the lens.

I also participated in retinal detachment repair surgery with Patrick Holmes Sellors and in dacryocystorhinostomy procedures with Hugh O'Donoghue ably assisted by my SHO, Peter Eustace who had just joined us from general practice at the time. All this activity, and highly efficient service to the patients, would not have been possible without the organisational and scheduling skills of the permanent chief secretary, Mrs. Sheila Tant and her office staff. It was also a great advantage to have the administrative staff office situated in the same building as the major outpatient department and not located in the general hospital secretary pool. This allowed for increased efficiency in the organisation of clinics and theatre lists. Mrs Tant's capability also involved the organisation of clinical conferences such as the annual Irish ophthalmological group surgical meetings, the South England Eye Surgery Soc. as well as many others scheduled from time to time. From the

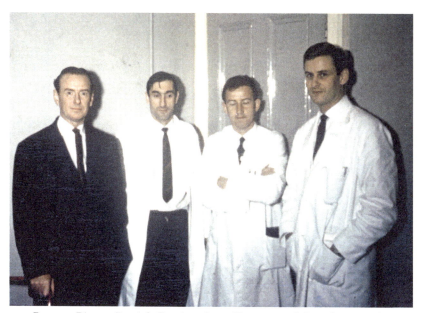

Dermot Pierse, Patrick Condon, Peter Eustace and Jonathan Kersley

accommodation point of view, I resided in the extremely convenient doctor's residence provided at Mayday Hospital. With the large growing population in the Borough of Croydon, the eye unit at Mayday General Hospital was extremely busy, with large numbers attending at outpatient clinics and augmented by the constant flow of emergencies to be dealt with.

The operating lists which were scheduled during the mornings, tended to clash with some of the clinics which meant that trying to be in two places at the one time, was quite wearing while also trying to supervise the work of the junior doctors who were less experienced. Working under this degree of pressure made the lunch breaks very welcome before starting the afternoon operating lists and extra clinics.

As the weather improved during the summer months, Peter Eustace my SHO, Maeve Ann Sandiford, the orthoptist and some of the juniors and myself, would often take a lunchtime break from the unit and go to the Crystal Palace National Stadium for a swim in the Olympic sized swimming pool which was open to the public at certain times and where one could also get a cup of coffee and a sandwich before heading back to work in the afternoon. This was great for the team morale of the unit and tended to relieve the pressure on us which was very intense some of the time.

As work was beginning to replace any degree of social life, I decided to join Streatham Rugby Club which was situated at the back of Mayday Hospital and extremely convenient for training and keeping some degree of fitness, ending up playing on the 3rd's team. It was also a great bonus from the social point of view in that every weekend, we were playing other London clubs such as London Irish and meeting up with other interesting Irish people from all walks of life.

Chapter 7
Learning the Art of Eye Microsurgery

International Microsurgical Study Group (IOMSG) 1966:
  As ophthalmic surgery advanced in sophistication, it became obvious to Professor Dr. Heinrich Harms of Tubingen and Professor Dr. Günter Mackensen of Freiburg, Germany, that the instrumentation required for this type of surgery had not kept pace with the degree of surgical progress. To promote research into this aspect of eye surgery, the IOMSG was set up by them with the first meeting at the University of Tubingen in 1966. At this meeting, presentations were made on improving visualisation during surgery using updated microscope design as well as changes in instrument technology. Major contributors to the group were Michael Roper-Hall from Birmingham and Dermot Pierse from Croydon. As surgical instrumentation became increasing important, the IOMSG increased in size attracting more ophthalmic surgeons to the group with subsequent meetings in Bürgenstock, Lucerne, Switzerland (1968), Mérida, Mexico (1970), Lund, Sweden (1972), and London (1974) the latter of which was organised by Dermot Pierse.

Dermot Pierse, MCh, FRCSI (1918–1995):
  Born in Dublin with a strong family medical background, dating back to his grandfather, Dermot was educated at Blackrock College and received his medical degree from the National University of Ireland, University College Dublin in 1941. He received his ophthalmic training at Bristol Eye Hospital and the Royal Westminster Ophthalmic Hospital, London. He became a consultant at Mayday Hospital in 1948 just prior to the start-up of the NHS, forging the development of the Croydon Eye Unit into a recognised training centre for ophthalmology. During his early

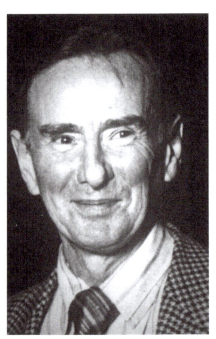

Mr. Dermot Pierse, FRCSI

career, as he became interested in attempts to improve the surgical instrumentation for modern cataract surgery, he was immediately attracted to join his fellow international colleagues in the IOM SG. Having an innovative and pioneering talent and extremely mechanically skilful, he set about modifying many of the existing instruments ophthalmologists were using at the time.

Dermot originally teamed up with an engineer to make the Pierse–Hoskins forceps design from stainless steel. This forceps embodied a notched tip principle of gripping tissue firmly without using the element of teeth which tended to crush and damage the delicate tissues of the eye and interfere significantly with wound healing.

He subsequently involved Derek Walter C Eng. M.I.E., with an aerospace background, who had engineering skills and manufacturing techniques working with Titanium Alloy which was a much lighter metal and less corrosive than stainless steel. Between 1966 and 1971, a variety of different forceps designs, a needle holder, a straight and angled fine scissors, a razor fragment holder, a diamond knife holder, and scleral support were manufactured. From 1971to 1974, Dermot set up a non-profit research group called MICRA Titanium Ltd., through which the following items were further developed: Diamond knife, Razor-Fragments, Fine cannulate, MICA cautery, Ophthalmodynamometer, Bifocal Binocular Microscope, MICRA micro surgical operating chair,

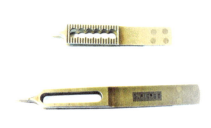

MICRA Titanium Forceps

Keeler Snake microscope, and Fibre optic illumination for use with surgical microscopes.

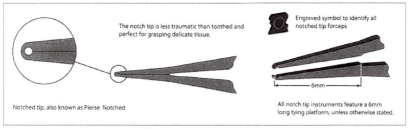

Pierse Notched Forceps

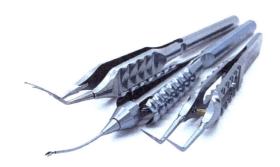

Pierse-Hoskins Forceps 300dpi

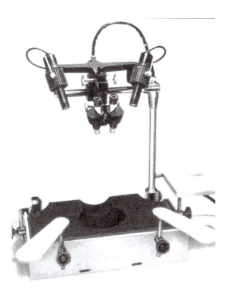

Pierse Keeler Operating Microscope System

In conjunction with the Keeler Optical Company, he started to introduce portable operating microscope systems that incorporated a headrest for the patient, its own fibre-optic lighting system, a binocular microscope, and armrests for the surgeon, all in one unit which could be easily transported and would fit on any operating table. With the daily continued use of the evolving operating microscope, Dermot's quality of cataract surgery in relation to wound architecture was fascinating to watch. Beginning with a

55

variety of bevelled, vertical and combined corneal and corneoscleral ab externo incisions, the final choice seemed to be a vertical corneal incision with pre-placed 10-0 nylon sutures to close the wound. This became the subject of a joint paper presented at the Oxford Congress and later published in the Transactions OSUK in 1968.[1]

By nature, he was a quiet person with little interest in casual conversation but with a mind that always seemed to be busy and somewhat disquieting to encounter. On the mornings of his outpatient clinics or operating lists, there was very little conversation, and silence was quite the norm waiting in the coffee room for things to start up and the work was in full swing. One of the most fascinating aspects of working with Dermot, was that he always had a standard type forceps or needle holder instrument that he had modified the night before at home in his workshop e, which he gave to the theatre staff to sterilise for him. This began with the Pierse-Hoskins forceps with the notched tips which were designed to replace the historically used toothed forceps, which he felt was more likely to damage tissues especially in relation to the surgery involved in corneal transplant procedures. Gradually newer designs of commonly used instruments started to emerge from his company MICRA Titanium Ltd, and other companies such as John Weiss, Duckworth and Kent and many others. This was particularly relevant in relation to the magnification issue, when for 20 years or more eye surgeons were using the standard head worn loupes and various types of goggles to visualise the minute anatomy of the eye.

As time passed, I began to become more comfortable with him as a colleague and not as a boss, in that I was able to discuss things as they cropped up. Whereas he was an excellent surgeon, he was more of an innovator with an enquiring engineering brain which I became to respect more and more. Apart from instrumentation, another issue which concerned him greatly and emanated from his work in corneal transplant surgery, was the constant search for improved suture materials, which up to then consisted mainly of 8-0 silk. This material was highly irritating for the patient postoperatively but had to remain in place until the wound had

---

1 Pierse, D, Condon, P.I.: "Cataract Sections Wound Closure" Trans. Ophthal. Soc.,UK LXXXXV11,41-420, 1968.

healed adequately. Unfortunately, whereas much work had been done by suture companies in relation to the larger materials used in general surgery, little had been accomplished by any company in relation to wound closure in ophthalmic surgery, there being a dearth of research with the newer types of materials such as non-absorbable nylon and polypropylene and other materials as used in general surgery.

Even though it was obvious initially that the much-reduced size of inert monofilament materials caused less inflammatory reaction particularly in corneal graft patients postoperatively there was very little hard evidence for this, and that further research would be required. We then started communications with Ethicon to make up a selection of single use 10-0 nylon/Prolene material attached to their needles which they subsequently supplied to us and which we reported on at the Oxford Congress in 1968.

Conference Organisation:

Whereas my first six months as a registrar working at Croydon could be considered a learning curve in many respects, little did I know that the following several months working there, would be even more of a learning experience. Whereas the surgical skills acquired in a programme for surgeons are an important part of their training, there are several other equally important managerial skills which are required when reaching consultant status. Not only do these involve administrative issues in dealing with staff and bureaucracy but apply greatly when it comes to the maintenance of standards for junior doctors in training.

This aspect of responsibility suddenly dawned on me when Dermot Pierse announced in February 1967, that he would be visiting the United States on a lecture tour in early March and had left Mrs. Sheila Tant, his chief secretary of the department and myself to organise the annual Croydon Surgical Course in his absence. Going on past courses that he had himself organised, these meetings involved the presentation of interesting cases, wet laboratory instruction in the use of surgical instruments and live surgery using closed-circuit television to demonstrate newer techniques with the newly developed surgical instruments including operating microscopes. A small trade exhibition and a modest social event for the delegates were also included.

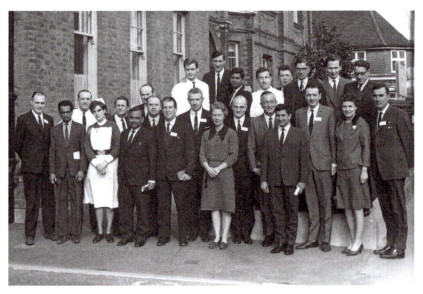

Irish Ophthalmic Surgical Study Group Croydon 1967

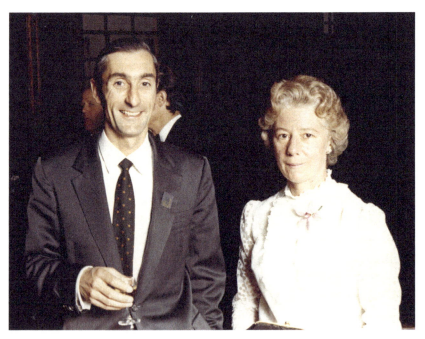

Conference Organisers Patrick Condon and Mrs. Sheila Tant

While the promotion of the meeting with printing of the programme and booking of the delegates, was taking care of by Mrs. Tant, the clinical program and arrangements for the meeting including the live surgery aspects and the CCTV fell to my brief. I was also being continually badgered by Dermot Pierse to look up scientific articles and material for his forthcoming presentations in the US. This was all done against an extremely busy background of daily outpatient clinics and operating lists. Whereas Mr. Patrick Holmes Sellors and Mr. Hugh O'Donoghue were extremely helpful in supplying some of the case presentations and in the live surgery sessions, for my part, I had to participate in active surgery carrying out a cataract and a glaucoma procedure under CCTV and a dacryocystorhinostomy under local anaesthesia which were organised at St. Anthony's Hospital where the surgical part of the meeting was held. The meeting, which was extremely successful, ran from the 2nd to 4th March 1967, and was attended by my father with his fellow colleagues from Cork, Limerick, Galway and several UK surgeons, who all enjoyed the meeting. This was followed a day later with a weekend visit by the seventy members of the South England Eye Surgeons group, which had been previously organised by Hugh O'Donoghue and involved case presentations and discussions on surgical problems and instrumentation. In Dermot's absence, my presentation of his corneal transplants case results, stimulated quite an active response from some of the attending Moorfields consultants

After all the excitement of the meetings had subsided, and the unit returned to normal, Dermot returned from his whirlwind lecture tour in the US, exhausted. Many of those he visited were very helpful to me in my first visit to the US later in 1970, when Dick Troutman offered me a Fellowship to work with him in the Downstate Medical Centre in New York subsequently.

With the experience gained in helping to organise and participate actively in the meeting, I felt a lot more confident in myself to take on more surgery which in the situation of long waiting lists for surgery, Dermot and his colleague consultants, were happy to allocate to m. As a result, I ended up operating four days a week, working with Patrick Holmes Sellors and Hugh O'Donoghue, on their patients and gaining greatly in experience. With cataract and glaucoma procedures routine for me, I also managed to operate on many retinal detachment repair cases, using some of the techniques taught to me by Eric Arnott a year previously in Surbiton. To complete my surgical experience, the only procedure I had not managed to do was a corneal transplant. Having assisted Dermot Pierse with many transplant procedures and worked with him using many different types of suture materials and techniques to stabilise the graft, together with the help of some excellent new products from Ethicon in the pipeline, I finally got round to doing my first corneal transplant before I left Croydon, which was extremely successful.

Dermot Pierse Academic Achievements:
– National University of Ireland (NUI) Extern Examiner in Ophthalmology: Dublin, Cork, Galway 1960s.
– President of the Ophthalmic section of the Royal Society of Medicine in 1982.
– Honorary Fellowship of Royal College Surgeons (FRCS) of Ireland in 1983.

Higher Qualifications:
As I approached the end of my year as registrar in Croydon in May 1967, I decided to take my three weeks annual leave to study for the London and Edinburgh FRCS and the National University of Ireland MCh examinations. Unfortunately, I failed the London examination which I found very difficult despite my surgical experience and was naturally quite disappointed. I did however continue to Galway where I took the MCh (NUI) exam under acting Professor Mr. Everard Hewson, with which I was subsequently conferred after the exam. I also went to Edinburgh where I sat for and successfully passed the exam for the Edinburgh Fellowship. As expected, the major emphasis of the exam was on neurology and neuro ophthalmology which involved a full neurological physical examination of a patient with multiple scattered demyelinating lesions as the clinical part, followed by a gruelling oral in which my knowledge from devouring David Cogans books and Frank Walsh Atlas, were severely tested.

Following these extremely testing times, I visited my parents at home in Tramore, Co. Waterford where I recuperated, running each morning on the beach to the sand hills and backs and fishing for shark with my father 12 miles off Dungarvan Head. While there, my mother had a photograph in her kitchen, of the University College Cork ladies hockey team featuring my two sisters and fellow teammate Dr. Ann Wall who I had dated a year previously in London for the St Patrick's Day Ball at the Dorchester Hotel and who I had kept in touch with intermittently since her return to her parents' home in Crookstown to study for her Primary FARCS exam in anaesthetics. While in Ireland, we arranged to meet in Cork before I returned to the Nuffield College in London for six weeks of intensive study in preparation for a repeat attempt to pass the London examination for the English Fellowship.

The Royal Eye Medical Ophthalmology Unit – Lambeth Hospital: 1967–1972

With the announcement by senior registrar, Joseph Walsh of his appointment to the Royal Victoria Eye and Ear and Our Lady's Children Hospitals in Dublin, the vacancy of the senior registrar post at the Medical Ophthalmology and Surgical Unit in Lambeth Hospital suddenly became available. As I have already mentioned, the Royal Eye department at Lambeth Hospital comprised an active surgical unit in which the consultants, senior registrar and registrar actively operated. It also housed the only purposely staffed Medical Ophthalmic Unit in the country. Ophthalmic consultants to the unit were Prof. David Hill, who succeeded the recently retired Prof. Arnold Sorsby, Mr. Alan Friedman and Mr. Noel Moores. The medical physicians appointed to the unit were neurologist Dr. Frank Clifford Rose, also at Queen Sq. Hospital for Nervous Diseases, cardiologist and vascular physician, Dr. Michael Harrington, also at the National Heart Hospital and Dr. Geraint James, physician for inflammatory disorders, also at the Royal Free Hospital, London. The purpose of the unit was to fully investigate patients with medical eye diseases in the fields of neuro ophthalmology, neuroendocrine, cardiovascular and inflammatory diseases involving the eye. The unit also had its own junior hospital staff who, at the time, were Drs. Michael and James Bowden, both with MRCP degrees, who arranged the admissions of patients for investigation to the unit and their case presentation, in conjunction with the eye senior registrar. At the weekly conferences decisions were made as to each patient's further management.

Whereas the posts of SHO and registrar in ophthalmology were held in rotation while passing through the Royal Eyre training programme, that of the senior registrar (SR) was regarded as a holding post for a consultancy in other hospitals as they become available. It was to be expected therefore that in the case of the SR post becoming vacant, there would be considerable competition for the position, for which I immediately applied. As it transpired, there was stiff opposition from four other well-qualified candidates, all with Fellowships. The only difference between the applicants happened to be the National University of Ireland (NUI) MCh degree with which I had recently been conferred, and because of which I was subsequently appointed in August 1967.

As my surgical ability and confidence had by now greatly improved thanks to the experience gained at Croydon, and with the FRCS (Edin.) and MCh (NUI) degrees, the consultants at Lambeth not only allowed me to assist them in surgery but gave me my own list of suitable patients on which to operate. In this way, I was able to increase my surgical expertise to other different procedures such as the repair of retinal detachments. In this respect Professor David Hill, who had been a consultant at Moorfields Hospital with Professor Barrie-Jones at the Institute of Ophthalmology in Judd St. and was particularly helpful. From the day he arrived, Prof Hill showed himself to be a highly dedicated hard-working conscientious consultant interested in high standards of surgery and patient care. Having worked with Mr. Lorimer Fison in the retinal clinic at Moorfields Eye Hospital, Prof Hill took on the retinal clinic at the Royal Eye Hospital appointing me as his chief assistant. At surgery, he was meticulous and extremely generous with his time and often assisted the registrar and junior doctors in their surgery. One example of this was when he assisted me doing a retinal detachment repair, in which he took me through each step of the procedure with meticulous care and attention which I greatly appreciated at the time. He was also extremely helpful with some of the complicated trauma cases.

My duties with the Medical Ophthalmology Unit involved the supervision of investigations and responsibility for the eye side of all patients admitted with medical, neurological, neuroendocrine and cardiovascular disease problems. Considerable experience was gained with Mr. A.I. Friedman, in the use of different instruments in the investigation and diagnosis of neuro ophthalmology, retinal and glaucoma visual field defects. Dr. Richard Huntsman, consultant haematologist at St. Thomas' Hospital, who had a particular interest in abnormal sickle cell haemoglobinopathies, also started referring patients to me for diagnosis and management of retinal problems arising in Jamaican patients attending his clinic. The ones with active eye problems ended up being seen at Prof Hill outpatient's clinic at the Royal Eye Hospital.

On taking up the SR post, I suddenly realised the increased responsibility of my position, and that one of my duties was to supervise the work of the junior SHO and registrar doctors in relation to the management of their patients and my responsibility to the consultants who were ultimately in charge. I also learned how to deputise work practices in the outpatient clinic to optimise the flow of patients and increase efficiency. Being first on call at night for eye emergencies covering the huge area south of the Thames, was at first a rather daunting task but gradually became one of a familiar routine. As SR doctors were expected to provide their own accommodation outside the hospital, I started looking at apartments in which to live and was lucky to be able to check in to the Middlesex Hospital residence hostel accommodation in Bayswater, where my good friend Dr. Conor Keane was living at the time. Facilities at the hostel suited me admirably in that it had a telephone answering service, a room service and domestic staff with breakfast provided each morning. From the social point of view, it was also conveniently located in an area blessed with good pubs and a good curry restaurant which Conor and I frequented.

FRCS Course Material Teaching Tutorials 1968-69:

With my unsuccessful attempt at the London FRCS exam in the spring, and the security of the SR post, I decided to retake the exam again in the autumn. To avoid a possible second failure, I decided that the best way to prepare oneself, for an exam of this magnitude, was to teach the subjects to others and encourage as much discussion as possible thereby learning from others. I subsequently set up teaching sessions each week for the junior doctors on the Royal Eye rotation programme, targeting the more difficult aspects of the various basic science subjects, such embryology, anatomy, physiology, and optics. As news got out about these sessions, we even had doctors from Moorfields Eye Hospital attend.

In my case, I applied to the Royal Eye Hospital board for 9 days study leave before the exam, which was initially refused, but grudgingly granted following pressure by the consultants. This enabled me to focus on aspects of the examination which I had found difficult on my first attempt. As a result of all these efforts, I finally passed the London FRCS Fellowship exam in November 1967. I was also delighted to learn that the three Royal Eye and four Moorfields doctors on our tutorials were also successful. As Christmas approached, I found myself on call with many emergencies to keep me busy and little time to celebrate my success. As to the New Year 1968, I also found myself on call but enjoyed the atmosphere and camaraderie of the staff at Lambeth in the build-up. I did however celebrate by visiting my favourite uncle and aunt, Philip and Alice Ianson who owned a pub in Warwickshire, for a weekend after all the festivities had died down. This was followed by consultant Mr. Noel Moores taking the junior staff and myself out to dinner in the West End and Prof. Hill and his wife inviting the juniors and myself, to his house on another occasion which was greatly appreciated.

Following a skiing holiday in Zermatt in early January 1968, I attended the conferring ceremony in the Royal College in Lincolns Inn Fields and was conferred with the Fellowship of the College in ophthalmology. Within a few months, I sat the FRCS exam in Dublin and passed the examination, thus completing the so-called "Triple Crown" of all exams.

Clubland Youth Club:

On considering my hospital responsibilities especially in relation to being on call for emergencies at night for the south London area, I decided to look for alternative accommodation in the Lambeth area and found out about a hostel on the Camberwell-Walworth Road not far from the hospital which occasionally took in students and supported a local boys club called Clubland.

Clubland Youth Club was an initiative set up by Methodist minister, Rev. Jimmy Butterworth before the war, designed to keep young boys in the area off the streets and was socially considered to be unique at the time. Whereas his church and accommodation for boys were destroyed in 1941 in the Blitz, his reputation and appreciation for his work, and that of his ministry, provided the impetus for a complete rebuild in the post-war period. This was funded totally by money raised in concerts at the London Palladium by Bob Hope with the support of actor Michael Caine, who grew up in this area and attended Clubland as a young lad. Following an interview with Rev. Butterworth and his wife, it transpired that there was some empty accommodation that was not being used and that I could rent on a temporary basis until I found more suitable accommodation.

Chapter 8
Medical Ophthalmology and Wound Healing Research

Royal College of Surgeons Wound Healing Research: Sickle Cell Eye Disease 1968–1972

With his strong background in research and the Research Department of Ophthalmology at the Roy College of Surgeons in Lincoln's Inn Fields, vacated by Prof Arnold Sorsby in 1966, Professor David Hill approached me about undertaking a research project at the RCS. With the Croydon background, a presentation at the Oxford Congress and a recent publication on cataract incision and suturing techniques, it was decided to investigate the feasibility of extending previous research by Gasset and Dohlmann, McPherson et al. and Richards et al. using more modern suture materials. Enquiries were then made as to the facilities for animal care at the College. A grant application was made to the South Western Metropolitan Regional Hospital Board for funding of the project which included the building of a tensiometer to measure the stress and strain of sutured incisions. With approval from the Department of Health, the animal welfare organisations, and the Royal College of Surgeons animal laboratory department staff, we set about planning the project which involved a supply of New Zealand white rabbits and their management in the college following surgery.

Surgical Techniques 1969–1972:

Following a year of administrative detail and further delays caused by problems of design and production of the tensiometer, I finally started the work in mid-1969. The anaesthetic consisted of an intravenous administration of an appropriate dose of barbiturate, followed by the surgery in which a Blumenthal anterior chamber maintainer connected to a continuous saline infusion was used to perform a preliminary extracapsular lens extraction. This was followed 3 weeks later by a second surgical procedure using the same technique, in which 4 separate full thickness incisions were made, one in each quadrant of the cornea, and each incision sutured with a different suture material, followed by inflation of the anterior chamber with air to prevent anterior adhesions of the iris to the posterior surface of the cornea. The animals were sacrificed at varying intervals of time after surgery, and each wound with its suture, was removed and subjected to both tensile strengths and histological assessment. Using a Zeiss Op Mic1 ENT microscope on a stand with a Beaulieu 16 mm film camera through a beam splitter, the behaviour of all incision specimens removed from the cornea of each animal, were photographed, and their breaking strains recorded by the tensiometer which was linked to a pen recorder showing specimen stress and strain on two separate channels.

A preliminary report of experiments comparing the effects of 6-0 plane and chromic collagen, 8-0 nylon and 8-0 virgin silk in corneal wounds in rabbits was made. Wound strength in the initial few days appeared to be proportional to the strength of the individual suture material with which the wound was stitched. With all but nylon, there was a fall in strength after the fourth day. By the twelfth day, all wounds except those stitched with

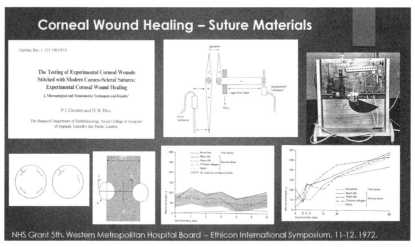

Modern Suture Materials Research – Methods

nylon were at their weakest, but thereafter there was a gradual increase in strength until at two months, it has reached a strength equivalent to 65% that of the original intact cornea. Wounds stitched with nylon, unlike those stitched with collagen or silk, showed a constant steady gain in tensile strength all the time. Histologically, nylon showed the least reaction, while collagen provoked the most inflammatory reaction. Virgin silk was the only suture material which seemed to encourage epithelial ingrowth along the suture track.

The project was best described in a film entitled "Corneal Wound Healing and Modern Suture Materials" and presented at a subsequent Ethicon International Symposium conference at the Royal College of Surgeons London in 1972. The results of the study were published in Ophthalmic Researc.5: 137-150 (1973).[2]

Acknowledgements were made at this and other presentations to: Mr. Ian Capperauld, FRCS. Medical Director of Ethicon and John Blythe, Representative who supplied the suture materials.

My Introduction to Sickle Cell Disease 1968:

While most of my duties were sited at the Lambeth, I used the facilities at the main St. Thomas' Hospital a lot and became quite friendly with a number of the consultants there, of which one was Dr. Richard Huntsman. He was a haematologist who was interested in genetics and whose clinic outpatients was largely composed of Jamaicans living in south London with a high prevalence of sickle cell variants. As many of these patients had eye problems and as the eye clinics at St. Thomas' Hospital were so busy with other problems, I managed to get Prof. Hill to allow me to see them at his outpatient clinic at the Royal Eye. Meanwhile, Dr. Huntsman's work with Professor Hermann Lehmann, author of "Mans Haemoglobins" at Cambridge University, proved to be invaluable in the classification of the different abnormal haemoglobin S variants (Hb S) in patients attending our eye clinic. The

---

2 Condon, P.I., Hill, D/W: "The Testing of Experimental Corneal Wounds Stitched with Modern Cornea - Scleral Sutures: Experimental Corneal Wound Healing 1. Microsurgical and Tensiometric Techmiques and Results".Ophthal. Research, 5:137-150,1973.

results of our findings were eventually published in the Journal of Clinical Pathology in 1972.[3] Little did I realise at the time, that sickle cell disease would eventually become a problem in Ireland due to the arrival of African immigrants carrying the sickle cell gene.

History of Abnormal Sickle Cell Hb S:

Since James Herrick in Chicago first described an abnormal looking red corpuscle as "sickle shaped", in a blood film of a dental student from Grenada in 1910, much research has been carried out worldwide to discover the effect of the Hb S molecule as the cause of sickle cell disease. In 1922, Dr. Vernon Mason of John Hopkins Hospital, Baltimore, described the first of four cases in the US which were all of African origin and was responsible for the term "sickle cell anaemia".

The relationship between sickle cell trait and the disease was elicited by two doctors working under different conditions, Dr James Neel in the Department of Genetics at Ann Arbour School of Medicine, US, and Dr. E. A. Beet, a colonial medical officer working in Zimbabwe. In 1940, both published that the disease resulted from the inheritance of the sickle cell gene from both parents and was the homozygous form. Reports then followed of an apparent sickle cell disease where one parent did not have the gene, and which led to the recognition of other abnormal haemoglobins, such as Hb C and Hb beta thalassaemia, that could interact with Hb S to produce symptoms. The next step in understanding was the use of Tiselius moving boundary electrophoresis which showed differences between Hb S and normal adult haemoglobin Hb A. This implied a difference of electrical charge and hence chemical composition of Hb S, prompting Dr. Linus Pauling to describe it as the first historical molecular disease in 1949. As investigating technology became more sophisticated, Dr Vernon Ingram and colleagues in Cambridge UK reported in 1957, that the difference in the background of Hb S, was the replacement of glutamic acid by valine at position 6 in the beta chain.

---

3 Blake, A. J., Condon, P.I., Gombels, B.M., Green, R.J., Huntsman, R.G., Jenkins, G.C. : "Sickle- Cell Haemoglobin C disease in London". Jour. Clinical Pathol.; 25, 49–55,1972.

Clinicopathological Manifestations of Sickle Cell Diseases:

One may ask how does this abnormal inherited haemoglobin affects health and cause widespread lesions throughout the body? In the normal person with red cells that contain normal adult haemoglobin (Hb A), the haemoglobin in the red cell picks up the oxygen while it is circulating through the lungs. On reaching the various organs throughout the body, it releases its oxygen to the tissues following which the normal red cell recirculates again to pick up more oxygen and the cycle repeats itself until the red cells are scavenged in the spleen after 120 days. In sickle cell disease, the same process is followed, but on releasing its oxygen to the tissues, the abnormal haemoglobin damages the red cell wall, the rupture of which results in the release of bilirubin pigment into the blood stream. This then puts more pressure on the spleen to scavenge the numerous red cell remnants which in turn leads to splenic enlargement and hypersplenism. The bone marrow attempts to keep up with the increased demand for red cells but in severe cases fails to do so, resulting in severe anemia. Other parts of the body affected are the kidneys with renal failure, the liver with jaundice and biliary stones, the long bones with severe bone pain from areas of infarction and when all of these happen together, a full-scale sickle cell crisis results. Whereas there are many other abnormal haemoglobins such as Hb C and Hb β-thalassaemia which can combine with the sickle cell gene, the disease conditions are much milder than the homozygous Hb SS form.

Chapter 9
Winds of Change 1968–1969

Waterford Hospital Eye Unit Locum:
With 18 months solid surgical experience, I felt reasonably confident to take on a locum consultant post for my father who was still actively working in Waterford. In April 1969, cataract operating lists and eyelid skin graft cases were scheduled for me by the theatre nurse, Sister Ryan. As I had already in the past seen my father operate on cataracts and marvelled at his dexterity using the Graefe knifeman ab internal procedure, which he performed flawlessly, as a son, I felt humbled to operate in his department. Bearing in mind the limitations of the surgical facilities at Ardkeen already outlined, I continued for the week carrying out some intraocular procedures on patients provided to me by Sister Ryan, avoiding only eyes and advanced cases, which for my level of experience and skill, were not appropriate. When not working in the theatre, I was busily employed seeing out patients both publicly and privately, which was a new experience for me.

In the space of time living at home, I enjoyed my father's company, fishing for salmon on the River Suir at Kilsheelan and a couple of drinks in the evening time after dinner. The slower pace of life compared to London, began to appeal to me and the photograph of Dr. Ann Wall in the Munster lady's hockey team with my two sisters, only encouraged me to further my friendship with her.

Wedding Bells:
It was the St Patrick's day in 1966, that I first invited Dr. Ann Wall from Crookstown, Co. Cork to celebrate our national feast day at the Dorchester Hotel while working as an SHO in Lambeth hospital. She happened to be working in the hospital

as a junior anaesthetist on the St. Thomas' Hospital anaesthetic rotations scheme and was recommended to me by a fellow colleague. In the following year, while returning home to see my parents and seeing her photograph in our house, I set up correspondence with her while working at Croydon as a registrar which continued into the following year with intermittent occasional meetings from time to time. These became more frequent when she returned to the Middlesex Hospital in London, where she worked as a registrar in 1968. During this time, we socialised together either with friends who owned a boat on the Thames or attending concerts in the Festival Hall. In September 1969, after proposing to her, we decided to get married and arranged the wedding for the 7th of February 1970 in Crookston. In the meantime, I had approached Rev. Jimmy Butterworth at Clubland as to possible accommodation for the newlyweds on our return to London. On explaining to him that both of us would be on call for our hospitals at night and weekends, with the need to be reasonably close to our work, he came up with a separate self-contained flat at the top of the building at Clubland which seemed to suit us at the time. On our return to London, both Ann and I were immediately plunged back into being on call and because we worked in different hospital settings, found difficulty in trying to coordinate a mutually compatible time off for a honeymoon. After six weeks, we eventually managed to slip away to the Dolomites fora skiing holiday in in Northern Italy.

USA Study Leave Tour and Jamaican Sickle Cell Project –1970:

With six years training in ophthalmology, including three in active surgery behind me, I applied for study leave to visit the major eye hospitals in the United States, which I had read about in those years. With this in mind, I approached Dermot Pierse and Prof. David Hill with a request for their references to undertake a study tour of some of the major eye hospitals and centres in the US. The project would involve the giving of presentations to the resident doctors in training at each centre visited on "Cataract and Corneal Graft Incisions and Suture Materials", and "The Prevalence of Ophthalmic Eye Problems in Sickle Cell patients in

London", while collecting information on the system of training in the US as compared to that employed in the UK. I then drafted an up-to-date CV outlining my training in ophthalmology, which I enclosed with letters to the various department heads of the hospitals I wished to visit. Those targeted were: Drs. Ed. Norton, Lawton -Smith and Don Gass at the Bascom Palmer Institute in Miami, Florida, Dr. Sam MacPherson, Raleigh, North Carolina, Prof. Edward Maumenee, John Hopkins Hospital, Baltimore, Drs. Austin Fink and Richard Troutman, Downstate Medical Centre, New York, the Ethicon facility in New Jersey, Dr. Malcolm McCannel in Minneapolis and lastly Dr. Pat O'Malley in South Bends, Indiana.

With encouraging replies from most of the US hospitals, I formulated an itinerary and applied to the South-West Metropolitan Regional Hospital Board for some help towards defraying my travel expenses for the visit and to the Royal Society of Medicine for a Keeler Award, both of which were successful. With full funding now well established, the Royal Eye St. Thomas' Hospital group were quite happy to release me for me for a two-month period of study leave without pay, while they hired an interim senior registrar to cover my absence. I had barely settled back in London after our honeymoon, when I received a request from Dr. Graham Serjeant, at the Medical Research Council Epidemiology unit in Kingston, Jamaica, with an invitation for me to visit with him to assess his patients with sickle cell conditions for manifestations of eye disease. It appeared that Dr. Huntsman had been visiting Dr. Serjeant and mentioned to him that I was planning a visit to the States, whereupon Dr. Serjeant requested that a visit by me to Jamaica might be included on the way there. Whereas Prof. Morton Goldberg in Chicago, had published widely on the more severe eye complications of sickle cell disease in black people in the United States, there was very little published work on the incidence of eye disease in the West Indian population. As St. Thomas' Hospital in London had a training arrangement for its doctors with the University Hospital of the West Indies in radiology, anaesthesiology, and orthopaedics, I made an application to the hospital group to participate in this study to be funded by the Welcome Trust out of Dr. Serjeant's Medical Research Council's budget.

Medical Research Council Epidemiology Unit, Kingston, Jamaica:

Following the foundation and building of the University Hospital of the West Indies (UHWI) in 1952, the Medical Research Council Epidemiology Unit was established on the campus at Mona on the outskirts of Kingston, Jamaica in the early '60s. The function of the unit was to carry out research into prevalent diseases such as malaria, diabetes, filariasis and others relevant to the Caribbean area. Dr. Paul Milner, consultant haematologist at the University Hospital, who had started a weekly clinic for sickle cell patients, was using electrophoretic techniques to categorise the variants and was in the process of collecting large amounts of data on these patients. Following a visit by Prof. Hermann Lehmann of Cambridge University, and author of "Mans Haemoglobins", to Dr. Milner's clinic, the consensus arrived at was that a unit at UHWI would be most suitable for further research into sickle cell disease.

In 1967, Dr. Graham Serjeant, who had been a senior registrar in cardiology at the Hammersmith Hospital in London, applied for a post in the Department of Medicine at the University Hospital of the West Indies and was appointed by Prof. Cruickshank, Prof of Medicine for a year, during which time, he carried out the usual duties looking after patients with varying medical conditions in the medical wards and its outpatients. During his year, Dr. Serjeant

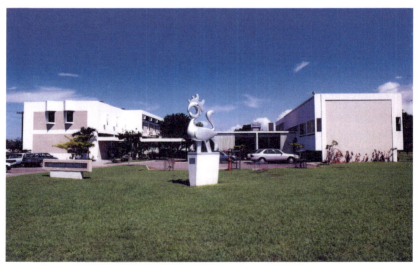

Medical Research Council Unit, UWI, Kingston, Jamaica, W.I

became acquainted with Dr. Paul Milner, assisting him in his sickle clinic while Dr. Serjeant's wife, Beryl, who was a fully trained laboratory technician, helped him with the laboratory work. During this year, on reviewing the potential for research into the clinical and genetic aspects of sickle cell disease, Dr. Serjeant applied to the UK based Wellcome Trust for a grant to investigate more thoroughly the extent and morbidity of the abnormal haemoglobins in the Jamaican population. This involved the setting up of a laboratory at the Medical Research Council Epidemiology unit, a central outpatients clinic in the Ripple Laboratory building on the campus of the University Hospital, a network of outpatient clinics at the various peripheral hospitals in the larger towns around the island of Jamaica, and a VW van equipped as a mobile clinic for locating and examining patients in the rural areas of the country. Following approval of the grant, Dr. Sarjent and his wife Beryl, implemented a medical sickle cell clinic service for the whole country of Jamaica, collecting massive amounts of data on the incidence of abnormal Hb S and the extent to which the disease incapacitated the Jamaican population.

After some time, realising that the research into abnormal haemoglobins was progressing rapidly from the scientific point of view, Dr. Serjeant and his wife, returned to Cambridge University to work with Prof. Lehmann in further studies of the involved abnormal genes. This was followed by a visit to the major units in the United States, which were also working on the molecular structures of abnormal haemoglobins. These contacts provided them with an international panel of experts, that served to expedite the Jamaican project. As a result, they became permanent members of the University medical community.

Leave Tour Begins Sept. 1970:

Having received many very enthusiastic and positive replies from Dr. Graham Serjeant in Kingston and the US ophthalmology centres to which I had written, my new wife, Ann and I, set off from London airport to Miami on the first leg of our journey. From Miami, we made the straightforward journey to Kingston with Air Jamaica, only to be greeted with a severe lightning storm as we landed at the airport. On disembarking from the plane, it was magnificent to encounter the lovely warm air and characteristic smells of the city as we looked forward to reaching our hotel. Unfortunately, this was not to happen, in that there was no one to meet us at the airport or any directions as to where we were staying. After several hours waiting at the airport for someone to collect us, we phoned the University Hospital of the West Indies enquiring if Dr. Sarjent was available, to be told that nobody knew of his whereabouts but that he was most likely to be at a country farm on the outskirts of Kingston, owned by a Mr. Robin Weiss and his wife Joan. Eventually having contacted Dr. Serjeant, we finally made our way to a small hotel in the Liguanea area of upper Kingston, not far from the University. On arrival at the hotel, having not eaten for some time, we found the local supermarket and with a couple of Red Stripe Jamaican beers, eventually got to sleep to await the next day fully refreshed. As it happened to be a bank holiday weekend, Dr Sarjent and his wife Beryl arrived and brought us up to the Weiss farm, where we enjoyed incredible typical Jamaican hospitality. The following day, Ann and I were transferred to an apartment on the campus of the University of the West Indies with a view overlooking the magnificent Blue Mountains. The campus itself was on the higher ground overlooking Kingston Harbour in the district of Mona, where most of the university staff lived and not far from the main Kingston city water reservoir area where many of the University staff used to run and exercise in the early morning. It was not uncommon to find oneself in the company of the Prime Minister, Mr. Michael Manley exercising in his training gear, before the temperatures rose excessively during the day. Following a period of settling in over the weekend, Dr. Serjeant, called by his first name Graham, introduced us to the staff at the Ripple building on campus with a view to setting up the equipment for the eye examination of his patients. Whereas I had brought my own indirect and direct ophthalmoscopes, the unit already had a Zeiss retinal camera with fluorescein angiographic capability that had been used for a previous diabetic study but very little else. The space in the Ripple building, which was designed for laboratory activities, had been adapted to provide a darkroom facility for examining eye outpatients which as we discovered very quickly, was not provided with air conditioning.

Meanwhile, Dr. Dinnick, Head of the anaesthetic department at the Middlesex Hospital in London, who had organised for Ann to work at UWI, introduced herself to her colleagues and was immediately allocated anaesthetic lists, one of which was Dr. Lockhart's eye list who we subsequently got to know.

Jamaican Sickle Cell Eye Disease Studies Begin:

By the time we arrived, Graham and Beryl Serjeant had accumulated a large group of patients with the sickle disease variants to be seen. These patients were made available for me to examine their eyes, which involved a quick vision test with an Ishihara test type plate on the wall at six metres distance, followed by the installation of mydriatic dilating drops into both eyes to expand their pupils for further examination. With fully dilated pupils, the patients would then have their eyes examined with the indirect ophthalmoscope to visualise the retina at the back of the eye in which the suspected pathology was located. A 360° examination of the peripheral retina, the optic nerve head and macula, all parts of the eye normally quite difficult to examine, was carried out on each patient. The discovery of eye conditions such as glaucoma or cataracts, were referred to the at UHWI general eye clinic for treatment. A hand drawing of each eye was recorded for each patient and in those with major pathology, a retinal photograph was taken with the Zeiss fundus camera.

As each patient could take at least half-an-hour for the eye check, the maximum number we could examine was about 10 in the morning and 10 in the afternoon. The team worked extremely well in that all the patients had a full general medical examination by Dr. Serjeant with blood taken by Beryl for haemoglobin

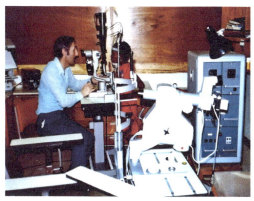

Retinal Photography of Sickle Cell patient in Ripple Building

and electrophoresis as part of their check-up. Whereas most of the patients with SS disease had just a mild degree of peripheral arteriolar shutdown in the retina with no major consequences from the sight point of view, some of the Hb SC's were found to have marked areas of vessel shutdown in the periphery of the retina with the formation of new vessels in the form of retinitis proliferates or "Sea-Fan" lesions, previously described by Goldberg in Chicago. These patients usually required a fluorescein angiogram to delineate the extent of the infarcted retina which necessitated an intravenous infusion of fluorescein dye followed by rapid sequential photographs of the retina as the dye progressed through the area. In some cases, the injection often caused reflex nausea and vomiting which had to be coped with at the time.

Unfortunately, the month of September in Jamaica happens to be the warmest month of the year and with little or no air conditioning in the Ripple building, it became quite intolerable during the day with temperatures combined with high humidity in the laboratory area, regularly rising to the '80s and '90s by midmorning. I, by this time, having usually had but a light breakfast, was thoroughly exhausted. However, with the addition of some oatmeal porridge for my breakfast, I discovered that I could make it till lunchtime, when the ingestion of a sandwich or goat pate assured me of enough energy to complete the day. As the month went by, I saw more and more patients with various aspects of the sickle cell variants which were all recorded and correlated with their haemoglobin type and patterns were beginning to fall into place. During this period, we collected lots of data and retinal photographs of some of these patients' eyes which we subsequently recorded in published work of the medical journals.

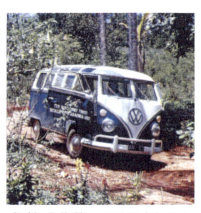
Sickle Cell Clinic VW Mobile Unit

When we were finished examining patients in the Kingston and surrounding areas, we carried out some clinics in Mandeville, Blackwater, and Montego Bay, where there were many more patients to be surveyed. To get to these clinics, we used the VW sickle cell van which could be darkened by inside curtains that allowed me to examine eyes. On one occasion the van penetrated the centre of a cane field to accommodate my examination of sugar cane workers. The wonderful thing about all of this, was being able to view the magnificent countryside of Jamaica and to experience the diverse and very friendly people we encountered in our travels. It was also very interesting to visit the different small towns and to meet with the doctors running the local hospitals in each area who had some incredible problems to deal with but great stories to tell.

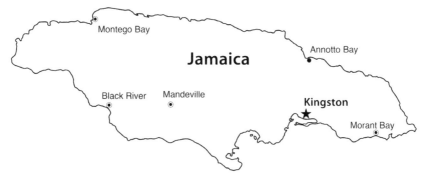

Island of Jamaica with Sickle Cell Clinics

During our month stayed in Jamaica, at weekends, Dr. Serjeant would occasionally lend us the VW van for us to travel around and get to know the area around Kingston, taking care to avoid downtown Kingston and the no-go areas. However, one of the attractions on the campus, was a lovely swimming pool where at weekends, we could sunbathe and socialise with the other staff working at the university. The other attractions in upper Kingston were the Liguanea Club with its swimming pool and squash court of which Graham was a member and would invite me to have a game of squash there followed by a swim, on a weekly basis. There was also a very nice Chinese restaurant called Mee Mees, which we also frequented with them at weekends. As the data was correlated at the end of each month, it was decided that our results should be published. We therefore put together three major papers on Hb SS, Hb S-Thal and Hb SC variants that were subsequently published in the American Journal of Ophthalmology in 1972, as well as a report of an unusual choroidal retinal degeneration in a case of SS diseases in the British Journal of Ophthalmology [4]. Careful documentation was also made of children with different variants, and patients with early signs of proliferative sickle retinopathy, with plans to review these patients in future visits for possible treatment.[5]

American Ophthalmology 1970:

Leaving my wife Ann in Jamaica to continue in the anaesthetic department at UHWI and the amenities and friendships developed during our time there, I departed in early October to Miami, finding local hotel accommodation close to the Bascom Palmer Institute, and presenting myself early the next morning to the chief resident at the Institute, who was expecting me. He had set up a day or two, for me to accompany him and his colleagues in their daily work which included attending outpatient clinics in the varying subspecialties and surgical operating lists. I was particularly interested in attending Dr. Lawton Smith's outpatient clinics who was one of the most well-known neuro ophthalmologists in the US. With a total of three years' experience of working in the Medical Ophthalmology Unit at the Royal Eye Lambeth, investigating neuro ophthalmology cases for Dr. Frank Clifford Rose, our neurologist, I found it fascinating to be able to discuss cases with him at the coffee breaks. As a man of deep faith, he exhibited an extraordinary kindness to patients in discussing their cases with them. Dr. Donald Gass, author of the "Stereoscopic Atlas of Macular Diseases: Diagnosis and Treatment" was also one of the doctors who I spent time within in his clinic. His expertise in retinal diseases and fluorescein angiographic investigating techniques, attracted patient referrals from all over the US, and his weekly case report sessions were incredibly fascinating to attend. I was also impressed by the quality of the resident junior doctors and had dinner with some of them to get to know more about their motivation and experiences of their training in ophthalmology at the Bascom Palmer.

Following a most successful visit to the Bascom Palmer

---

4 Condon, P.I.C., Serjeant, G.R., Ikeda, H. "Unusual Chorioretinal degeneration in Sickle Cell Disease". B. J. Ophthalmology: 57: 81-88;1973.

5 Condon, P.I., Serjeant, G.R. "Ocular findings in children with sickle cell disease in Jamaica". Br.J. Ophthalmology: 57:644-649; 1974.

Institute, I rented a car and drove from Miami to Raleigh, North Carolina along the eastern coast highway, stopping off at various places like Daytona Beach, to experience, for the first time what America had to offer. As I drove north through South Carolina, I was enthralled by the beauty of the Appalachian Mountains and arrived in Raleigh where I located Dr. Sam MacPherson's surgery. Dr. MacPherson was a member of the International Ophthalmic Microsurgery Study Group (IOMSG) and well known to Dermot Pierse for his research work on cataract surgery and the designer of the McPherson forceps used in corneal transplant surgery. He was therefore quite interested to hear of my proposed studies with Prof. David Hill at the Royal College of Surgeons in London. During my visit there, as well as watching some very beautiful transplant work by Dr. MacPherson and his team, I gave my usual presentation to the residents.

My next stop was the Johns Hopkins Hospital in Baltimore, where I reported to Prof. Edward Maumenee's office, who subsequently introduced me to the chief resident, and the resident staff and scheduled me for my presentations to be given during the clinical rounds and presentation of cases at their weekly meeting. My presentation on cataract and transplant incisions and suture materials seemed extremely relevant for those resident doctors starting surgery and lots of questions were asked of me regarding aspects of technique. Being a big city with a large black population, the talk on sickle-cell eye disease with comparisons of London and Jamaica with Baltimore, provoked much interest also. At one stage during my visit there, Prof Maumenee in an early morning meeting, offered me a part-time research project funded privately if I wished to relocate to the US.

Having never been to New York before, the experience of arriving in Manhattan was most inspiring. Dr. Austen Fink introduced me to Dr. Richard Troutman, both of whom worked at Downstate Medical Centre in New York. Both also had private practices in different areas of the city, with Dr. Austen Fink living and working in Brooklyn which was very fashionable at the time. Both were anterior segment surgeons, Dr Fink developing a special irrigation aspiration push pull cannula for aspirating lens material in paediatric cataracts. On the other hand, as a member of the IOMSG and well known to Dermot Pierse, Dr. Richard Troutman was very much involved in the development of operating microscope design for eye surgery. While in New York, Dr Austen Fink and his wife Selma looked after me at their home in Brooklyn while my presentations were made at the Downstate Medical Centre where I met the residents. It was at this time, that Dr. Troutman offered me a fellowship in corneal transplantation, to which I almost committed myself at the time, but with reservations to consider it on my return to the UK.

Having been in touch with the UK Ethicon company in Edinburgh regarding a request to visit the permanent headquarters in Somerville, New Jersey, I took the opportunity while in New York to visit the facility to see how the sutures and needles we were using in ophthalmic surgery were made. Being purely a manufacturing plant, without any ophthalmology staff present, my talk on wound healing with different suture materials was of little interest.

It was at this time, that Ann quit her anaesthetic locum in Kingston to come to New York to join me in Austin and Selma Fink's house in Brooklyn and from where we enjoyed sightseeing in Manhatten and attended a concert by Errol Garner at the that Central Park Hotel. Our next journey was purely a social one to visit Dr. Terry O'Callaghan and his wife Eileen and their children in Connecticut which we reached by train from New York. The O'Callaghan's who got married before emigrating to the US some years previously, were friends going back to our school days in Clonmel. Terry was a pathologist who for a period had been in the US army and was currently working with a pathology group servicing hospitals in a large area of the state of Maine. Terry had organised a campervan for the four of us to take a trip up country to Vermont to see the autumn colours and enjoy the scenery which turned out to be magnificent and a great break from the work intensity of the previous six weeks. After enjoying the company of the O'Callaghan's and their children in Connecticut, we then made our way to Boston from where Ann returned to London.

I then journeyed on to meet up with Dr. Malcolm McCannel in Minneapolis, famous in ophthalmology for the McCannel suture, who had developed a new highly efficient patient record system in his office practice, which had been highlighted at the Annual American Academy of Ophthalmology conferences and highly rated. I finally concluded my tour by visiting Dr. Patrick O'Malley in South Bends, Indiana, whose brother Dr. Conor O'Malley in Chicago, independently of Dr. Robert Machemer, had developed a vitreous cutter and irrigation system for carrying out vitrectomy procedures in eyes with severe vitreoretinal problems. The O'Malley brothers, sons of surgeon O'Malley, at Galway University Hospital, emigrated to the States, and eventually became ophthalmologists. My interest in visiting Pat O'Malley, was to gather some spin-off information on the latest in vitrectomy techniques with these cutters. As Prof. Hill was performing most of the retinal detachment work at the Royal Eye Hospital in Lambeth, and as vitreo-retinal surgery had not yet evolved, I felt that some update information would be of interest to him on my return. As this was my final port of call, the time had come to leave the US and return to the UK to resume my senior registrar post. On my return, I completed a full report of the Jamaican and US visits, to the SW Metropolitan Hospital Board and the Keener Award sponsors at the RSM which Dermot Pierse and Prof. David Hill were extremely happy with.

On my return to the UK, I initially found it quite strange to be back at work and on call for emergencies at night, but I was glad to be back at base in our apartment in Clubland, at 54, Camberwell Rd., south London. During the next few months in 1970, while still working as a senior registrar, with Prof Hill, Alan Friedman and Noel Moore at the Lambeth / Royal Eye and the Medical Ophthalmology Unit with physicians Drs. Frank Clifford Rose, Geraint James, and Michael Harrington, I started the rabbit research work at the College. To get the rabbit project off the ground, Prof Hill organised for me to have a day a week put aside from my normal hospital schedule.

Meanwhile, Ann who had returned to work at the Middlesex, found herself pregnant with our first child and decided to quit work and help me with the rabbit work which we started in the run-up to Christmas 1970. Despite being on call for Christmas at the end of a telephone, Ann and I celebrated the Christmas festivities with the Butterworths, enjoying their friendship and our apartment in Clubland and going to visit our very best dental friends, Ita and Thorough O'Brien, in Barnes, West London for Christmas and St. Stephens Day. While 1971 got off to a great start with the anticipation of a baby on the way, new developments in health services in Ireland were beginning to emerge.

UK NHS Consultant Post 1971–1973:

As time went by, and with our first baby due in April 1971, it became obvious that we had to decide on a place in which to establish a permanent place of residence. With my research beginning to take off well and increasing confidence in myself as a surgeon and organiser, I realised that for the sake of our future family, I would need a more secure position, so that when I was approached by the St. Mary's NHS hospital group based at Sidcup, Kent in relation to a consultancy in ophthalmology at Bromley and Farnborough general hospitals, I applied for the post. On attending for the interview, I was pleasantly surprised to be appointed along with another candidate, Dr. Ross Lewis from Scotland after which I subsequently resigned my position as senior registrar to the Royal Eye/St. Thomas' group. However, with my ongoing corneal wound project at the Royal College to be completed and my continuing interest with Dr. Huntsman's sickle-cell patients seen at the Royal Eye, I was offered an honorary consultant post at both institutions to allow me to continue with these projects.

Whereas Bromley Gen Hospital was a small general hospital situated in the middle of Bromley town, Farnborough hospital was much larger and situated in more attractive countryside. Both hospitals were administered from the larger regional St Mary's Hospital in Sidcup. Having resigned from the Royal Eye Lambeth group in late 1971, I started work in both hospitals with my new colleague Ross Lewis, both of us taking over from our predecessors Drs. Ruston and Lyle in late 1971. Surgical facilities and inpatient beds were provided at Bromley as part of a general surgery and casualty department, while outpatient clinics were scheduled for both hospitals. Having both come from senior registrar posts in major ophthalmic training centres independent from general hospitals, having to share operating theatre space with general and emergency surgery was foreign to us. However, without any other alternative, we endeavoured to start our surgical lists as separate sessions beginning with extraocular surgery first. Within a short time however, the occurrence of a series of Pseudomonas Pyocyaneus infections in general surgical cases, combined with cross infection in the general wards in which the eye patients were recovering, alerted us to the possibility of post-operative endophthalmitis which after an intraocular procedure, could have serious consequences. Quickly plans were developed for the provision of a separate emergency casualty operating theatre with clean air ventilation to augment the existing surgical unit and to postpone intraocular surgery pending this development. To offset these difficulties, the facilities at the outpatients' clinics were improved with some new equipment and extra nursing and optometric help in the provision of a more efficient service. With a period of surgical stalemate, the available time was spent maximising the research work at the College with my wife Ann, helping me with the anaesthetics for the animal work. On these occasions, without the facility of a babyminder, Ann was forced to bring our daughter, Fiona with her, parking her under the Prof's desk in his office while we got on with the work in the laboratory, popping out at intervals to feed her. Unfortunately, this arrangement did not last very long when we discovered that Ann was pregnant with our second child, Richard who was born in May 1972. This provided me with the impetus to complete the wound healing project at the college and to correlate and publish the results with Prof David Hill. While waiting for improvements in theatre facilities for eye surgery in Bromley, and with a new daughter, now almost a year old, we decided to leave the flat at Clubland in Camberwell Road and rent a house in Biggin Hill.

With the completion of the new casualty theatre and adjoining facility separate from the general theatre inpatient area, Dr. Lewis and I, feeling more comfortable from the legal point of view, started intraocular cataract surgery and dealing with surgical emergencies. With the facilities to provide a safe surgical environment, and the potential for developing a private practice, we moved house to Orpington where our second child was born in 1972. It was while living here that Dr. Richard Huntsman from St. Thomas's Hospital loaned us his mobile home on the Broads in Norfolk for a weekend where we brought our daughter and our young son Richard who was still in nappies. As it turned out to be the wettest Bank Holiday on record, with floods surrounding the mobile home, and children banned from the local pubs, we ended up returning to Orpington with bags of dirty nappies and soaking wet clothes. It was during this final damp interval that the final discussions with the South Eastern Area health board in Ireland were conducted.

Seismic Health Changes in Ireland:

In 1966, in Ireland, a new Health Bill became law followed in 1970 by a government White Paper transferring health from local authorities to regional health boards. In 1971 a year later, eight area health boards were formed with agreement to upgrade the services in each health board area by establishing regional general hospitals with adequate consultant cover to develop by 1975. Unfortunately, my father who was diagnosed with a carcinoma of the lung and wishing to enjoy some retirement, resigned his position as consultant ophthalmologist to Waterford, and Dr. Peter Doherty was appointed as locum in his stead. The permanent post was advertised by the local appointments committee (LAC) in Dublin and I immediately applied for the post. Our decision to return to Ireland was now made. I attended for the interview at the local appointments office in O'Connell St. Dublin in the summer of 1971. The interview was conducted by the secretary and chairman of the board and was followed by a separate mandatory test in the Irish language.

Area Health Board – Department of Health Negotiations 1971–1973:

Following the LAC interview, I received a letter from the newly formed South East Area Health Board (SEAHB) general hospitals manager, Mr. George Bourke in September 1971, informing me of my successful appointment and welcoming me to the SEAHB. In response to this, I immediately replied, pointing out that the existing unit with one surgeon, one theatre nurse and a single operating room doubling up as an outpatient and casualty clinic area, when not used for surgery, was originally planned for the county of Waterford and surrounding area with a population of approximately 100,000. In my letter, I outlined certain recommendations in line with a future service for five counties and the population which at that time was between 350,000 and 500,000. Included with this recommendation, was information from the Irish Faculty of Ophthalmology regarding the standards required for a regional eye unit of this size and that three consultants and a backup nursing staff would eventually be required. I also added details of the increasing demands and requirements anticipated by the Connelly Child Health Services Report (1967) in which 13.1% of children have a visual defect and 3.4% amblyopia and the need for orthoptic services to manage them. But most of all, the urgent need was for a proper serviced operating theatre with adequate facilities for safe intraocular surgery for patients.

It transpired that my documentation was then put before the SEAH board itself for their approval before being submitted to the Department of Health (DOH), following which I received a letter from them in January 1972, accepting the need for these requirements, but suggesting a postponement until the service had been established and the requirements properly assessed.

In May 1972, I was informed that the basic equipment for the unit was approved except for a few items which the DOH felt should be left until the unit was up and running and demand created for their use. As regards the surgical theatre unit, contractual arrangements were going ahead but nothing completely confirmed. In August 1972, I sent a detailed resume of the extra staff that would be required to provide a regional ophthalmic service with details of my current UK and University of the West Indies commitments for the following period and requesting study leave for me to fulfil these commitments before returning to Ireland.

However, by this time my father had developed secondary spread of his cancer which was responsible for severe pain that required inpatient treatment at the Matter Hospital in Dublin, and I decided to visit him there.

Almost at the same time, I received a request from the Department of Health, located in the Custom House in Dublin, to attend a meeting there to be chaired by the Secretary of the Department at which the Chief Medical Officer, Dr. Alphie Walsh would attend. Having visited my father who was responding well to the treatment, I went to the meeting at the Custom House, to be faced with rather a large interview board of about ten people with a lady as chairperson. After the usual pleasantries from the various members including Dr. Walsh with whom I had already met and discussed the necessary upgrades, the meeting proceeded, the main question being as to when I would be prepared to take up the post. My immediate response was to refer to the documentation that I had sent to the SEAHB regarding the upgrading of the existing unit to make it safe for major intraocular surgery and to provide the necessary staffing for it to function professionally. After explaining everything to the board, it was explained to me that there was some degree of urgency in having the post permanently filled. I then asked the yet unspoken question, as to whether they had the funding to carry out the theatre work, to which the lady chairperson replied that the costings for the project had just been approved. I was then asked the same question again as to when I was ready to start. Having been reassured by this board in the Department itself, I had no other option but to accept the post and agree to a starting date of December 1973.

On 19th October 1972, a letter from Mr. Bourke confirmed that all aspects of my requirements had been approved by the DOH and their wish for me to give them a date to take up the post. I finally received a letter in January 1973, reassuring me about approval for the equipment, the staffing, and the surgical extension to the unit and demanding a starting date. On 8th February 1973, I received a letter from personnel manager, Mr. JP Quinn on behalf of the SEAHB confirming my appointment by the board from 12th February 1973 with study leave without pay from 12th February to 30th November 1973 and with a commitment to take up actual duty on the 1st of December 1973. With the future of our family finally committed to returning to Ireland, I prepared myself by finishing off my various commitments to St. Thomas' and the Eye Research with Prof Hill at the Royal College and offered my resignation to the NHS Kent office and St Mary's Hospital in Sidcup in mid-1973.

MRC Jamaican Sickle Cell Project Renewal April–May1973:

In the meantime, Dr. Graham Serjeant was in contact with me, about the patients in whom we had discovered active retinopathy that needed treatment and wanting me to return to the unit in Jamaica for this purpose. Being on study leave without pay from the SEAHB and with travel for me and accommodation for our family while in Jamaica provided by the MRC, I decided to take the opportunity to return there. Whereas I travelled on my own from London, my wife and two children travelled from Crookstown in County Cork via London directly to Kingston. On arrival there, Graham had arranged for us to have a small apartment on the UWI campus with a local Jamaican lady to help Ann with the children.

Whereas the work was very similar to that of my previous visit, I did have the opportunity to also examine a wider age group of patients, ranging from children to elderly patients with various forms of sickle cell disease which provided significant information as to the progression of these conditions.[6]

However, the prime object of the visit was to treat the patients with the growth of abnormal new retinal vessels, some of which had already started to bleed internally into the vitreous.[7] These lesions, located internally at the edge of the retina, could only be diagnosed with fluorescein angiography and in shape resembled a well-recognised coral found generally in the Caribbean Ocean and originally named "sea fans" by Goldberg in Chicago. The method of treatment involved the closing down of the feeder arterial blood supply to these abnormal blood vessels, with a powerful focused light beam using a photo coagulator instrument which was loaned from the manufacturing company and shipped to Jamaica for the project.

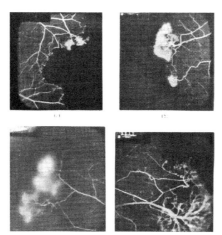

Potential for Retinal Haemorrhage – Proliferative Retinopathy

---

6 Condon, P. I., Gray, R., Serjeant. G.R., "The Progression of Sickle Cell Eye disease in Jamaica".Doc. Ophthal.: 39: 203-210; 1975.

7 Condon, P.I., Serjeant, G.R. "Photocoagulation in proliferative sickle retinopathy: Results of a 5 Year Study.". Br. J. Ophthalmology: 64:832-840,1980.

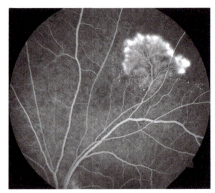
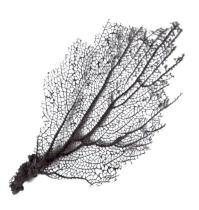

Sea Fan Neovascularisation *Actual "Sea Fan" Coral – Name for Proliferative Sickle Retinopathy*

During my time there, as my commitment to the SEAHB was not due to start until the end of 1973, and with free accommodation while in Jamaica, we decided to extend our time there after the research project at the University was completed, and to a have a holiday exploring the beauty of one of the most picturesque islands in the Caribbean. Part of this involved several days stay in a holiday resort on the north coast called Goblin Hill, in the area where Fleming wrote the James Bond series of books and possibly one of the most beautiful parts of Jamaica. It was also an opportunity for us to visit Dunn's River Falls and to boat ride down the magnificent river cascading down from the mountains to the sea at Ocho Rios.

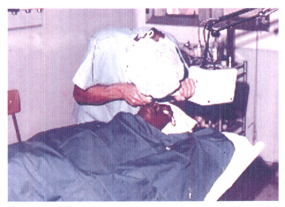

Photocoagulation of a patient with active retinopathy

Domestic Issues:

On our return to Ireland, Ann and the two children travelled on to Crookstown, where they stayed with Ann's parents, while I stayed with my mother, visiting my father who was still in hospital with deteriorating health. Without delay, I began looking for a house for us in which to live and finally bought No. 4, Parnell St., just off The Mall in the centre of Waterford. While I was still able to use my father's practice house to see private patients at 128, The Quay, the idea was to live and practice privately from the house in Parnell Street eventually. As the Parnell Street house was purely a residential house that was never previously used for commercial reasons, I set about modifying it to accommodate a family of four persons on the upper floors with a medical practice on the ground floor. This entailed gaining planning permission for a dormer extension on the top floor, installing a kitchen on the first floor and modifying the ground floor to incorporate a secretary's office and a doctors consulting room. This was all done with the help of builder Mr. William Fewer, who carried out the work on the top floor replacing the existing slate roof with a flat one and providing the house with a top flat which increased the accommodation available for the family. As to the family living room area, much of the internal work was carried out by me in the early hours of the morning before going to work and after work in the evenings. Unfortunately, my neighbours next door ran a bed and breakfast establishment, and on one occasion reported me to the police for "disturbing the peace". This resulted in me facing the Garda squad car with a warning concerning the noise and its disturbing effect on my neighbours' guests. It was around this time, that I decided to leave my mother's accommodation in Tramore and moved myself into Parnell Street and work from there. The refurbishment of the house being now complete, Ann left her parents' home in Crookstown and moved into Parnell Street, where we continued to live for the next few years and where our sons Edmond and Jonathan were subsequently born.

Chapter 10
The Building of a Regional Eye Healthcare Service. The Importance of Integration 1974–1976

Management:

The perception of ophthalmology as a specialty in the science of medicine, has always been regarded as a minor one by the medical profession and in the minds of the public, medical doctors specialising in ophthalmology, are often confused with opticians in the testing and provision of glasses. However, in the minds of those who provide medical services to the public, the provision of services that provide and maintain the quality of sight and restore vision, has always been regarded as a priority. To this end, the introduction of the Health Bill to integrate services generally provided an excellent opportunity for the various aspects of ophthalmology to be integrated with greater continuity of care. The fact that the SEAHB had separate general managers for the different services located in the same building as the CEO at their headquarters in Kilkenny, was to be a great asset for the ongoing development of the eyecare services in the southeast of the country. To this end, it seemed essential to me that to provide a comprehensive ophthalmological service to the public in this area, there had to be an approach involving three sectors of individual services, namely hospital, community care, and paediatric services.

Hospital Services:

The Eye department at Ardkeen Hospital in Waterford, occupying an old sanatorium single storey building and operating for 15 years since 1959, was difficult for me to get used to, half of which was allocated to ear nose and throat surgery with the other half for ophthalmology. The ophthalmology section consisted of three 6 bedded wards, a kitchen, toilets and one large room in which outpatients and casualty patients were seen, but which also doubled up as an operating theatre for surgical procedures. To avoid intraocular infections post operatively, this area had to be thoroughly disinfected and prepared with equipment and a small steam sterilising unit prior to each operating list. All operating theatre gowns, patient drapes and large instruments were supplied in pre-sterilised drums supplied by the Central Sterilising Supply Department (CSSD). The unit was staffed with a Moorfields Hospital eye theatre trained sister who managed the running of the unit. In December 1973, I took over as consultant from Mr. Peter Doherty, who had been doing a locum for my father for some time. With no junior staff, I immediately found myself on call 24 hours a day, seven days a week (24/7) with my father in the final stages of illness, hospitalised in Ardkeen. On arriving in Waterford, my first calls were to my two colleague ophthalmologists working in Waterford for some time, Dr J. Louis Ryan and Dr. Paddy Prendiville. Louis Ryan had worked with my father and had his MCh degree in ophthalmic surgery and was in private practice in Parnell Street and Kilkenny. Paddy Prendiville was the official ophthalmologist to the factory at Waterford Crystal. As well as practicing privately in Catherine Street, he also held outpatient clinics both in Waterford and Dungarvan. As a single ophthalmologist for an area as large area as the south-east, I approached Louis Ryan as to whether he would be prepared to act as locum for me at the hospital during my vacation time off and to assist me with some of the clinics. I then consulted the health board for sessions for him to do at the hospital and to reimburse him when on duty for me during vacation periods. Bearing in mind the enormity of the task in front of us, the health board agreed to his part-time participation in the services of the unit which obviously was a great support to me as the services expanded exponentially.

 As there was a significant backlog of surgical patients to deal with, I immediately started working with two operation lists a week, which included urgent cataracts and glaucoma patients which were mostly done under local anaesthesia and some squints using my good friend and anaesthetist Dr. John Mitchell who had been doing the eye lists for my father for some time. Emergency surgery was carried out in the same room using Dr. John Shanahan, consultant anaesthetist. Because of the simultaneous use of the operating room as an outpatient clinic on non-operating days, and the limited access for eye casualties to be seen during operating sessions, a separate small casualty room was set up in the paediatric unit of the hospital which could always be used around the clock without any inconvenience to the main unit.

Community Care Eye Services:

As my contract involved the provision of ophthalmological services to the five counties of Waterford, Kilkenny, Carlow, Wexford, and South Tipperary, with a population of approximately 450,000 at the time, I was anxious to expedite not only the provision of surgical services but also to attempt to coordinate the community care aspect of ophthalmology in the area. To this end, it was necessary to involve the managers and individual directors of community care in the SEAHB and attempt to coordinate their organisational activities such as eye outpatient clinics with the hospital services. At the time, there were several non-surgical medical ophthalmologists practising in the South-Eastern area who as well as providing eye testing and the provision of spectacles to patients under the Sight Testing Scheme, were also looking after medical eye problems. These problems included conditions such as diabetes, glaucoma and children with visual defects such as short-sightedness or myopia, and eye conditions such as squint and amblyopia. Many of these doctors were working with temporary contracts for the SEAHB in the local medical services with little contact with the central unit department. To facilitate the delivery of ophthalmic care throughout the area and obviating the need for patients to travel to Waterford, I also agreed to personally attend the most needed clinics at the time, which were the James Green community care facility in Kilkenny, and the ones at Carlow St. Dymphna's Hospital and St Joseph's Hospital in Clonmel. To integrate them further into a general ophthalmological service for the area, I negotiated with the health board that each practitioner would attend a clinic monthly at the central unit in Waterford, working with me and bringing patients for second opinions that were of concern to them. Part of this arrangement was my availability to them for telephone consultations. Wexford at the time were extremely fortunate to have Dr. Aidan Ryan and his wife Monica providing excellent medical ophthalmology and optical dispensing services in the Wexford–Enniscorthy area.

Inclusion of General Practitioners:

In an effort to coordinate the services throughout the southeast, it was essential that the general practitioners of the area, be involved and aware of the ophthalmology services being put in place in Waterford and the individual peripheral clinics in their areas. As most major towns in the various counties already had local clinical societies composed of general practitioners, medical directors of community care and healthcare workers, these societies were extremely helpful in the dissemination of information regarding the services we were about to provide. I proceeded to notify general practitioners in each area of the arrangements, providing them with instructions in techniques of eye examination and giving them lectures on eye problems such as "The Red Eye" and other basic conditions that could help when treating their own patients with such problems. The ophthalmic activities in Waterford with details of a referral system for problems they might encounter in their surgeries were disseminated to all.

Children's Eye Testing Scheme – Breaking the Backlog:

While the health boards children's sight testing screening service in which trained nurses measured the visions of children attending schools, was very efficient, the referral system to the eye medical ophthalmologist for testing for glasses, was extremely slow with large waiting lists. The main reason for this was the shortage of medical ophthalmology doctors to do the testing and the relatively small numbers who they were able to test during each average 2 to 3-hour clinical session. These delays in the appointment system for testing were also accentuated by having to use pupil dilating eye drops and to wait for the pupils to dilate, before being tested. There then followed further delays in the children having to wait to see the dispensing optician contracted by the health board to dispense glasses for them on the prescription from the medical ophthalmologist. This was then followed by a period before the doctor could see the child again to check the vision with the glasses and diagnose any degree of amblyopia or lazy eye which might then require treatment, possibly with a patch. On reviewing the logistics of the situation, it seemed that the process could be speed up by sending out a prescription for the eye dilating drops to the parents beforehand with instructions to instil the drops sometime shortly before the clinic. This would enable the doctor without delay to immediately test the child for glasses using a recognised dynamic retinoscopy technique (Amer. Academy of Ophthalmology), and with an indirect ophthalmoscope immediately perform a screening examination for any conditions affecting the retina or optic nerve. A prescription for glasses and an appointment for the dispensing optician would then be given to the parents. It was also felt that all children with their new glasses would then be subsequently reviewed by the schools' nurses and children with defective vision were referred back to the ophthalmologist for further management.

Having consulted with the clerical staff in the Kilkenny and Carlow areas, regarding sending out prescriptions for the drops and tighter booking of the clinics, I decided to take on the project personally participating with the clinic nurses and secretaries. We soon discovered that the possibility of testing 6 to 8 children per hour, was feasible which included the giving of a prescription for glasses to attend the optician. With just one session a week, a noticeable reduction in children awaiting sight testing was evident, resulting in the system being extended to the other eye clinics successfully. The problem then of course was for the nurse at the school's clinic to see them again with their glasses for a further vision check and referring any child with defective vision to be seen by the eye doctor for possible patching for a lazy eye or a surgical squint procedure to straighten the eye. While there was some opposition at first in initiating this policy of working, the appointment of an orthoptist was considered a priority. The reduction in the waiting list backlog resulted in many children having their eyesight restored and their appearance improved, a blessing that would last throughout their lives.

Establishng Children's Squint Services in the Southeast:

The condition of squint in children whereby one eye goes out of alignment with the other, can be an indication of an underlying visual defect which needs to be corrected as early as possible in the child's life with suitable glasses. Failure to do so, can result in total blindness in one eye for the rest of the child's life, a condition called amblyopia. Treatment consists of an eye test for glasses to correct any degree of short or long sightedness, followed by patching of the good eye to make the weak eye with poor vision recover.

Assuming the incident of squint in children would be the same as in the UK, and because of the large numbers of children per family unit in Ireland with one third of the population under the age of 12 years at the time, it was to be expected that there would be about 1,655 children with manifest squints per 100,000 of the population in the country. Bearing in mind that many of these children with squints require surgery to straighten their eyes from a cosmetic point of view, I found it important at the time to review the services in the south-east for these children.

After considerable discussion with the Programme Manager, and the Directors of Community Care of the individual counties in the south-east, it was decided to implement the already published previous Minister for Health's 1967 Connolly Child Health Services Report.[8] This included an overall incidence of 13.1% visual defects and 3.4% incidence of squint in a non-randomised series of 51,780 schoolchildren with the following recommendations:

> "An adequately equipped central clinic in each county; the introduction of an appointments system at clinics; changing from the present contract system of supplying spectacles to one based on more personal services; extension of orthotic services for the treatment of squint; more routine ophthalmic surgery at regional level; minor ophthalmic surgery at local level and greater utilisation of ophthalmic beds at Limerick Regional Hospital and Ardkeen Hospital, Waterford".

---

8 Connolly Report (1967): Government Publican Sale Office. Dublin (Prl.171).

Having worked with orthoptists in London, I wrote an article for Irish Medical Journal that was subsequently published entitled "The Place of Orthoptics in the Provision of Squint Services in Ireland".[9] The result was to get immediate approval for the funding of an orthoptist to be employed by the SEAHB. Within the following months, a Ms Beatrix Haskins, with a Diploma in Orthoptics (DO) was appointed.

Paediatric Surgery Ardkeen.
Clearing the Backlog 1974–1975:

With the increased development of the services from the incorporation of the various outpatient clinics in the SEAHB and the referrals from general practitioners, waiting lists for surgery increased dramatically with many demands building up at the unit in Waterford. For instance, with the provision of a 24/7 eye casualty service, more and more accidents and emergencies were being referred. With the acquisition of Ms Beatrix Haskins, orthoptist to the area in 1978, and the breaking of the waiting list backlog for eye testing and subsequent screening for surgery, there developed a huge increase in the number of children awaiting corrective squint surgery. In fact, not to compromise the accident and emergency side of things and the routine surgical lists in the unit, a temporary separate surgical and anaesthetic recovery unit was opened in the end ward of the Regional Paediatric Unit, in Ardkeen Hospital to facilitate squint surgery on children.

The system involved two operating tables side-by-side with two anaesthetists working while I alternately operated on each child with no more than short interval breaks to allow for a change of gown and gloves. The use of the beds in the paediatric ward was essential for this exercise, the children being discharged from hospital the following day. This extra service provided by the hospital was greatly appreciated by the children's parents who were extremely pleased after waiting years to have their children's eyes straightened and the stigma of their social unacceptability restored.

---

9 Condon, P.I.: "The Place of Orthoptics in the Provision of Squint Services in Ireland". Editorial Irish Medical Jour. Vol. 73 1.3,1980

Faculty of Ophthalmology and Irish Medical Organisation:

On my return to Ireland, to acquaint myself with Irish medical politics, I joined in quick succession the Irish Faculty of Ophthalmologists, the Irish Ophthalmological Society and the Irish Medical Organisation. Whereas the Faculty comprised mostly of out of Dublin ophthalmologists with one or two from the Eye and Ear Hospital, the IMO represented all medical professionals and was the official negotiating organisation in dealings with the Government and the Department of Health. With the implementation of the area health boards, and the process of regionalisation, the working practices of consultants in the hospital's services were changed and in some their contracts upgraded. For doctors working in community care, especially for ophthalmologists, little had changed. At the various Faculty meetings, it became obvious from the ophthalmic medical practitioners practising outside the hospitals, that many of them had no proper contracts of employment and were being remunerated for their work on a part-time basis without any degree of permanency and most certainly without any guarantee of a pension. Also, it was only when we started involving them in our clinics at the hospital and attending some of their clinics in the community, that we discovered the appalling conditions that these ophthalmologists were consigned to work with in their local areas. In many cases, the locations for the eye clinics were situated in totally ill-equipped GP dispensary buildings with nothing more than a box of eye testing lenses, a loupe for magnification examination of the eye, an ophthalmoscope, retinoscope and a poorly illuminated cardboard test type suspended by a nail in the wall, and most of the time at an incorrect distance from the patient.

The Sight Testing Scheme and Charles J. Haughey Minister for Health 1973–1979:

The Sight Testing Scheme was introduced by the government in 1980, allowing accessibility to the medical profession to test and prescribe glasses for patients with a medical card. Whereas optometrists were allowed to dispense glasses to those with medical cards, to my knowledge, they were not remunerated for prescribing, which was unacceptable to them. As a result, Gerard Brady, of Brady's Opticians, located in Minister for Health's,

Charles J. Haughey's constituency, canvassed Mr. Haughey to bring about changes that would allow optometrists the privilege of both prescribing and dispensing glasses to medical card holders. With representations from the IMO over conditions of service for medical eye doctors, a meeting with the Minister in his office in the Department of Health, on the top floor of the Bus Arus building opposite the Custom House, was arranged. Subsequently, a delegation of ophthalmologists headed by Noel Reilley, CEO from the IMO, attended his office in a large room with a huge desk, behind which was a door covered by a curtain. Arriving late, Mr Haughey entered through the door from behind the curtain and stood there without a word, eyeballing each one of us, one by one silently. Then sitting down at the desk before speaking, he addressed us with "Well, gentlemen, what can I do for you". In contrast to the usual welcoming words at interviews to make visitors feel comfortable, Haughey obviously, with his manner, was out to intimidate us which I discovered afterwards was a typical ploy of his when he wanted the meeting to go his way.

The discussion started from our side in which we outlined the necessity for a medical examination of eyes when being tested for glasses, which was currently being provided by medical practitioners and that optometrists without a medical training, were not qualified to diagnose serious medical illnesses, such as brain tumours and abnormal retinal and optic nerve conditions at the back of the eye. In return, Mr. Haughey indicated that from his knowledge, optometrists receive lectures from the medical profession in their training about these conditions and that he would have no objection to them becoming involved in the scheme. We also objected to the use of pharmaceutical eye drops by optometrists for the purposes of examination of children which we felt should only be prescribed and administered by suitably qualified medically persons. Despite these arguments across the table with Mr. Haughey, it was concluded by him that optometrists should be admitted to the scheme as it was far more convenient for members of the public to attend their local optometrist than having to travel to a clinic to have their eyes tested for glasses.

The next part of the interview concerned the conditions of work for medical ophthalmologists operating outside the hospitals and the equipping of the eye clinics throughout the country which we described in detail to him and with which he was suitably impressed. It was obvious in his reply, that he had already been in contact with various area health boards and was extremely aware of the failure to provide proper contracts of work for ophthalmologists employed by them. He immediately replied to the problem indicating that medical ophthalmologists working in a temporary capacity, could quite easily be incorporated into the newly introduced area health board existing community care system on a salaried permanent basis, with which our delegation was extremely pleased and which eventually transpired. It was also agreed that optometrists be allowed to participate in the prescribing of glasses for medical card holders.

Working with Architects and Builders:

I had barely started operating in the old eye department at Ardkeen, when I received a phone call from a Gregory Egan of the architect's firm, Lardner and Partners in Dublin, requesting a meeting to discuss the extension and modifications of the building required to the existing sanatorium block and the rehousing necessary to continue with the service while in construction. It seemed that Lardner and Partners had been given the contract to rebuild the new regional hospital and were working with a Swedish firm of architects with this in mind. Having sent a number of alternative designs to George Bourke, programme manager for general hospitals, it did not take very long to draw up a plan for the facilities that needed to be incorporated into the building programme, one of which was to include a clean-air laminar flow system for the theatre area and a pre-stressed concrete roof to support a ceiling mounted Zeiss operating microscope for intraocular surgery in the main operating room. In order not to disrupt the existing surgical and outpatient services, a separate surgical unit extension at the end of the building was considered the most convenient way in achieving the necessary required facilities. This would allow the existing unit to remain intact with its existing services until the new extension could be opened and interconnected with a small corridor. In relation to the outpatient's area, it was decided to build a small T shaped extension off the existing entrance to house the secretary's office, two consulting rooms, a large orthotic room, and a small casualty area without compromising the existing bed numbers in the unit.

Within six months, by July 1974, we were running three operating lists per week, one general and two special outpatient clinics in glaucoma and retinal diseases in conjunction with Dr. Louis Ryan, all within the existing accommodation.

For a period of two years from 1974 to 1976, the new operating theatre complex continued to be built without any major disruption to the existing services. During this period, several nurses were sent for specialised eye theatre training course at Moorfields Eye Hospital in London, one of which was Ms Rita McGinn. Several other nurses, specially delegated to the eye department, who received their Ophthalmic Nursing Diploma (OND) qualification at the Royal Victoria Eye and Ear Hospital in Dublin, also returned to Waterford as staff nurses, becoming involved in the specialised eye nursing care of inpatients and outpatient's clinic work. Despite the relatively restricted facilities for surgery at Ardkeen, we still managed to carry out 591 major eye operations in the 12-month period from January to December 1975.

Chapter 11
The Building of a Regional Eye Healthcare Department of Ophthalmology

The official opening of the Waterford Regional Eye Unit was marked by a meeting of the Royal Academy of Medicine in Ireland (RAMI)-Ophthalmic section and opened with the Croydon Lecture by Mr. Dermot Pierse entitled "The Correction of Aphakia". At a reception and dinner at the Ardree Hotel, Minister for Health, Mr. Brendan Corish, officially opened the unit to the public. A full days scientific programme was followed the next day by a visit to the unit where a cataract and squint procedure were carried out using the high definition Hitachi closed circuit

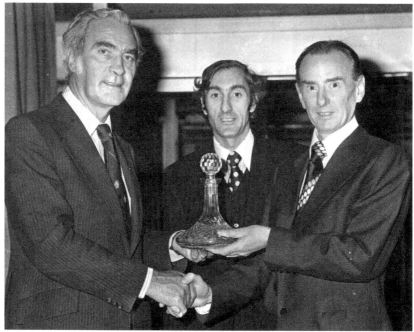

Official Opening of New Ophthalmic Surgical Theatre Unit by MOH in 1976

television system and interesting post graft patients of mine were discussed. The meeting was closed by Prof Desmond Archer, President of the RAMI.

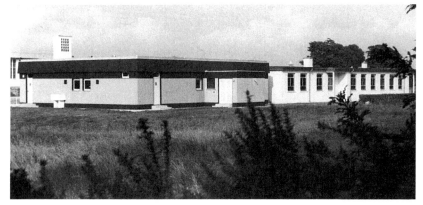

New Ophthalmic Surgical Theatre Unit Ardkeen Hospital 1976

ROYAL ACADEMY OF MEDICINE IN IRELAND
SECTION OF OPHTHALMOLOGY

President - Professor Desmond Archer

The Section of OPHTHALMOLOGY will meet in the Ardree Hotel, Waterford on Friday, September 24th and Saturday, September 25th, 1976. The Meeting will be held in conjunction with the Croydon Lecture to be given at the inauguration of the South Eastern Regional Eye Unit, Ardkeen Hospital, Waterford.

A G E N D A

September 24th
6.30 p.m.   The Croydon Lecture: "The Correction of Aphakia"
            Dermot Pierse (London)

8.00 p.m.   Reception and Dinner

September 25th
9.30 a.m.   "Evaluation of a New Electric Tonometer"
            Patrick Condon & J.L.Ryan (Waterford)

            "Future Prospects in Bio-Medical Engineering"
            Mr. Jack Hoskins (London)

            "Virus Keratitis"
            L.M.T. Collum & Geraldine Kelly (Dublin)

            "Unusual Lesions of the Lacrimal Apparatus"
            Yvonne Canavan & Peter Gormley (Belfast)

10.45 a.m. Coffee

11.15 a.m. "Photo Coagulation in Diabetes"
            Hung Chang (London)

            "Delivery of Drugs to the Eye"
            John Nolan (Galway)

            "The EMI C.A.T. Scanner and Orbital Tumours"
            Maurice Fenton & Anthony B Smith (Dublin)

            "Problems associated with Abnormal Blinking
            with particular reference to Contact Lenses"
            Jonathan Kersley (London)

12.30 p.m. Visit to Regional Eye Unit, Ardkeen Hospital (Waterford)

2.00 p.m.   Reception and Lunch
            (Courtesy of Ethicon Ltd., Edimburgh)

                                    G.P. Crookes,
                                    Sectional Secretary.

Royal Acad. of Medicine in Ireland Conference 1976

Period of Development 1976–1982:

Having taken almost two years to complete while we were working in the old unit, there was an air of complete excitement and elation as we started our surgical lists in the new environment complete with a new Zeiss operating microscope system, a wired in CCTV system and piped anaesthetic gases for the anaesthetists as well as a patient's recovery room. The separate instrument sterilising area was also a great bonus for the nursing staff in the preparation and sterilisation of the delicate ophthalmic instruments that we routinely used and recycled between cases. Separate changing rooms for the staff entering the theatre area were also available to maintain relatively sterile conditions within the surgical area.

Complicated Cataracts and Glaucoma procedures:

While routine cataract and glaucoma surgery were being done, more advanced cases demanding increased operating microscopic facilities were carried out. The standard cataract procedure at the time was an intracapsular lens extraction using Chymotrypsin and cryoextraction with occasional use of anterior chamber Rayner Intraocular Mark IX1 angle supported lens implants.

Retinal Detachment and Photocoagulation:

The acquisition of the Zeiss retinal camera with fluorescein angiographic capability and the use of a portable photo coagulator for treating diseases of the retina, in theatre and outpatients, was vital in the treatment of internal haemorrhages within the eye especially in relation to the large numbers of diabetics attending the clinics.

Glaucoma Visual Field Testing:

The extra room allocated to the glaucoma technician for visual field testing and for provocative water drinking testing for raised intraocular pressure and its measurement, proved to be invaluable in the diagnosis and management of glaucoma.

Contact lens Fitting:

The fitting of contact lenses in children after congenital cataract procedures was essential for the restoration of sight postoperatively and for those patients who at the time could not have a lens implant and were intolerant to the wearing of extremely thick glasses.

Orthoptic Squint Clinic:

The addition of a special room for the orthoptist to interview children with visual disabilities and squint problems in the company of their parents, was a major advance in the extension of the new unit. The use of special equipment in the management of squint involving special exercises to help and restore vision was vital.

Surgical Efficiency:

In the six-month period between January – July 1976, 560 surgical procedures were performed almost the same as carried out in the whole year before in the old unit.

Junior Hospital Doctor:

With the increasing help of the ophthalmic medical practitioners in the peripheral outpatient clinics and my colleague, Dr. Louis Ryan with the glaucoma and retinal outpatients in the unit, I was well able to cope with being single handed and on call 24/7. After several months in service, we suddenly began to notice a slow increase in casualty attendances at out of hours times, some of which were pretty horrific injuries and which had to be surgically dealt with as emergencies. Having no junior staff at the time, I applied to the board for a junior SHO to be appointed to deal with clerking the admissions for surgery, assisting at the clinics and operations and being on call for emergencies at night. Without any difficulty, a post was advertised. As a junior doctor post in ophthalmology in a nondescript unit down the country, was not a very attractive post to apply for, my expectations of filling the post were not terribly high. So it was fortuitous that at the time, my younger brother, Richard, who had just finish an SHO job in Dublin and was awaiting a post in the UK, was able to take up the SHO job in Waterford. He subsequently stayed with us for a year before he moved onwards to an SHO post position in Moorfields in London in his chosen speciality of ophthalmology. During his stay with us, a child was admitted having sustained a serious eye injury as a result of being hit by a golf ball. During the night following his admission, the child lapsed into a deepening coma. Richard accurately analysed the situation and had the child transferred to the care of surgery for treatment of a subdural haematoma, an undoubtedly life-saving accomplishment.

As the reputation of the units began to grow as a training centre for ophthalmology and recognised by the colleges, we continued to appoint junior hospital doctors on a six-month to one-year bit basis. Whereas these doctors all received a good basic training in practical diagnostics and minor eye treatments, facilities were made available to them for time off to travel to Dublin to attended the talks by consultants at the Eye and Ear Hospital and courses in optics organised by Mr. Hugh O'Donoghue, consultant ophthalmologist at the Mater Hospital in Dublin, who was a great help to them when it came to the Diploma examination.

Extra Consultant:

While it was a great relief to have some help at last, it was obvious from the severity of some of the injuries that were showing up in casualty, we would definitely need another consultant especially with an interest in trauma. By this stage, having now been a lone consultant working 24/7 for 5 years, I applied to the SEAHB for a second consultant with a medical retinal special interest which they willingly agreed to, and which was advertised subsequently in the usual journals.

Vitreoretinal Surgery:

It was great pleasure for me to be told that Dr. Philip Cleary, from Tipperary, was at the time training in vitreoretinal surgery at the Doheny Institute in California, US, and was interested in the post. Following the usual interviewing process, Philip was appointed and started work in November 1978.

Standard retinal detachment surgery involves operating on the outside of the eye using a silastic plastic material to buckle the sclera inwardly towards the detached retina. This approximation then allowed the retina to reattach itself to the sclera thereby sealing the hole in the retina. Vitreoretinal surgery involves microscopic keyhole type surgery within the eye to work directly on the retina. This type of surgery was developed by Robert Machemer in the US in the early '70s for retinal detachments due to internal traction on the retina following haemorrhage into

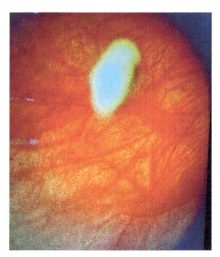

Fig 1. Steel splinter retained inside the eye – Hammering Injury

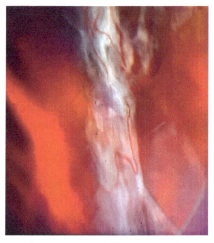

Fig 2. Vitreoretinal fibrotic membrane in a diabetic

the vitreous such as occurs in diabetics, and intraocular infections. The technique is also used for the peeling off from the retina of fine surface epi retinal membranes, the sealing of macular holes, and the draining of subretinal haematomas, which can now all be successfully treated with this technology.

As one of the first surgeons in Ireland to offer vitreoretinal capabilities using the newly introduced Ocutome vitreous cutter and specially designed microsurgical instruments for operating inside the eye, he soon started to receive patients with advanced retinal detachments and severe eye injuries from other centres around the country, such as these patients, one with pieces of steel embedded inside the eye (Fig.1) and severe diabetics with advanced retinal detachments from fibrosis of the internal structures due to bleeding (Fig.2).

Union Porters Work-To-Rule:

On the 9th October, 1980, I returned to Ardkeen from Cashel Gen Hospital, with eyes donated by a patient who had died as the result of a road traffic accident and started my operating list which I finished at 2 PM. My colleague Dr. Cleary was ready to start his afternoon list but there was no patient present. The transporting porter was apparently on an extended lunch break in the boiler house. On enquiring into the situation, we were informed that there was a picket on the eye theatre because of some labour disruption. Dr Cleary and myself, with the help from the staff transported the patient to and from surgery which resulted in our eye theatre being blacked listed by the union. Unfortunately, the situation was further aggravated with the corneal transplant procedure using the corneas donated earlier that day. Whereas we had no portering assistance within the unit, the oxygen cylinders which were on the outside of the building were allowed to be replaced. Further action was then taken by the porters union to inhibit further theatre work by refusing to transport the soiled operating theatre linen to the laundry, resulting in the staff and myself taking it home to wash and bring back the following day for further operating lists. While we continued to work without any porter assistance, a picket was them placed outside the gate and nursing staff were then prohibited from bringing their cars into the hospital campus, having to leave them on the road outside. Eventually the dispute was settled between the management and the union and the porter in question was allocated alternate duties.

Third Consultant Appointment:

Taking notice of the services the SEAHB were providing in the south-east, Comhairle na nOspideal in its "Discussion Document – Development of Hospital Ophthalmic Services" (1981), outlined the need for a third consultant appointment to the Regional Eye Department at Ardkeen. Mr. Aidan Murray was subsequently appointed to the unit in October 1981. Meanwhile, in an attempt to increase the input of ophthalmology at Cork University Hospital, Prof. Denis O'Sullivan, Professor of Medicine at UCC, offered Mr. Cleary a position there with funding for a separate surgical unit, and the prospect of a Professorship in Ophthalmology at UCC. Philip accepted the position and subsequently departed in October 1982. In April 1983, Mr. Aidan Murray also resigned to take up a consultant post at Cork University Hospital. Both consultants were replaced by ophthalmologists with special interests. While both trained as general ophthalmologists, Dr. Peter Tormey specialised in paediatrics and Dr. Patrick Hayes specialised in in medical retina and vitreoretinal surgery.

Second SHO Post:

From 1976 to 1986, the new theatre and outpatient facilities at Ardkeen were providing full-scale ophthalmological inpatient, outpatient and emergency casualty eye services to approximately half a million people. The increase in the volume and complexity of the surgery and outpatient attendances with three operating surgeons, put considerable pressure on the one single handed junior doctor whose job involved the medical examination of all admissions for surgery, attendance at operating lists and outpatient clinics as well as being on duty for eye emergencies at unsocial hours. Because of the apprenticeship nature of the post in working under close supervision with the consultants, the junior post in Waterford was highly regarded and recognised for training by the Royal College of Surgeons, which attracted quality applicants every time the position became available. It was during this period, that we were responsible for the training of doctors from India, Pakistan, Italy, Iraq and other countries all of whom returned to their countries of origin to continue their professions and subsequently keeping in touch with us many years later.

In late 1983, Dr. Margaret Pierse joined us as a junior hospital doctor with little or no experience in ophthalmology. As a lady with great determination and single-mindedness, she worked extremely hard to build up a competent level of expertise extremely quickly and without any difficulty passed her DO examination. As the only junior doctor on call for emergencies at night and working during the day assisting at outpatients and clerking in the patients for surgery, she soon found herself working around the clock. In an attempt to relieve her situation, all three consultants helped by offering to stand in on call at night, which in many situations resulted in one of us having to operate on serious accident cases. There was also the problem of replacing Dr. Pierse with her degree of expertise on her time off, with juniors most of whom have little or no ophthalmological experience.

It was at this point, that we approached the SEAHB for a second SHO in ophthalmology to allow Dr. Pierse her allocated time off and study leave for which she was entitled. With little or no response for several months, we enlisted the services of the Irish Medical Organisation to apply pressure in favour of the extra post. After several months of inaction, in May 1985, we had no other option but to reduce services to a level consistent with professional safety for patients. On further explanation to management on the detailed hours of work, the legal responsibility involved and the realities of the situation, the second SHO post was finally approved.

Chapter 12
Modern Cataract Surgery – The Beginning

**Pioneers in Lens Implant Surgery 1970s
and Extracapsular Cataract Surgery:**

Whereas the technique of removing the cataract from the eye varied over the years, it was only following the meticulous research by UK ophthalmic surgeons Drs. Harold Ridley and Peter Choyce and Dutch surgeons Drs. Cornelius Binkhorst and Jan Worst, that the concept of inserting an artificial lens into the eye after removal of the cataract was finally accepted. The method by which this was done was to retain the capsule of the original lens and its attachments after the cataract has been removed and to insert the implant into the capsular bag left behind and locate it behind the pupil. This was then called the extracapsular technique and is the current standard operation carried out today all over the world.

Cornelius Binkhorst (1912–1995) best known to his many friends and colleagues affectionately as Kees, more than any other, was responsible for the development of successful long-term lens implant surgery. He also championed the return to extracapsular surgery to stabilise the lens implant and dramatically reduced the complications rates of retinal detachment and late corneal decompensation. Kees was born in Rotterdam in the Netherlands and graduated from the University of Leiden in 1939. He spent 3 years in specialised eye training at the University Eye Hospital there. He practised in Terneuzen, located in in the most remote corner of Holland, as he would say. Its remoteness was not a barrier, however, to the stream of colleagues, admirers, and disciples who came to learn from the master. Binkhorst studied Ridley's method in London and made significant contributions in the preparation of lenses so they would be non-toxic to the eye. Between October 31st, 1955, and January 31st, 1957, Binkhorst inserted 16 Ridley lenses. Although 10 of the 13 eyes, with a follow-up of at least 21 months, had 20/40 vision or better, Binkhorst concluded that the use of the Ridley lens demanded 'too much of the human hand'. He then implanted 35 rigid anterior chamber lenses and 38 Danheim lenses. Although much easier to insert, he had grave reservations about anterior chamber lenses for the rest of his career because of the problems these early lenses caused. He then developed the four-loop iris clip lens in 1957 and implanted the first one on 11th August, 1958. Having noted an inadvertent displacement of the anterior loop of the four looped lens into the posterior chamber with obvious increased protection of the cornea, he purposely removed the anterior loupes cautiously and so gave rise to the modern extracapsular fixated lens implant on September 16th, 1965.

By 1971, Binkhorst was advocating extracapsular surgery. For him this was not a change in technique, since he had done extracapsular and intracapsular cataract surgery throughout his career, but rather a change in emphasis. The stability that the extracapsular extraction had on the iris clip lens located behind the pupil, was found to dramatically reduce late corneal decompensation. It also reduced the rate of retinal detachment, due to reduced endophthalmodonis, a term that Binkhorst coined to help explain the advantages of the extracapsular technique. He also kept meticulous records and reported his results with extreme openness and honesty. A very thorough analysis of his pioneering work is available in Nordlohne's landmark thesis "The Intraocular Implant Lens" (W. Junk BV the Hague, 1975), which he himself published with 70 other papers. Binkhorst was a founder of the International Intraocular Implant Club and its president from 1977 to 1980. He was

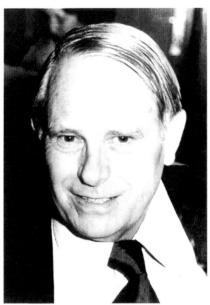

Dr. Cornelius (Kees) Binkhorst (1912-1995)

president of the Netherlands Dutch Intraocular Lens Implant Soc. from 1977–1980; and president of the European Intraocular Implant Council from 1980 to 1987. In 1975, the American Society of Cataract and Refractive Surgeons Society inaugurated the Binkhorst Medal Lecture and made Kees the first recipient. He was an early recipient of the of the International Intraocular Implant Clubs Ridley Medal and the Charamis and Cross medal. He was an honorary member of the American, French, German, The Nederlands, and Canadian implant societies and received the freemen of the city of Terneuzen.

When he began lens implantation, he was told sternly by his colleagues in the Dutch Ophthalmological Society to stop. In recognition of his enormous contribution to cataract surgery and the visual rehabilitation of patients by successful developments of the lens implant, the same society later awarded him the prestigious Snellen medal. Both personally and professionally, Kees was remarkable for his openness and modesty. The reverence with which his colleagues held for him never affected his humility. Following a stroke 1991, he subsequently passed away in 1995.

United Kingdom Intra Ocular Implant Society (UKIOIS). Cataract Surgery Developments 1977:

UKIOIS was formed in Dec 1976 with Drs. Neil Dallas, President (Bristol), John Pearse, Secretary, (Bromsgrove), and Piers Percival, Treasurer, (Scarborough) with a Council consisting of Eric Arnott(London), Walther Rich (Exeter), Hung Chang (Cambridge), Peter Choyce (Southend on Sea), Alan Ridgway (Manchester), Michael Roper-Hall (Birmingham), and myself Patrick Condon (Ireland) with Rayners representing the implant industry. As the aim of the society was to promote implant and cataract surgery, surgical workshops were set up at centres throughout the country beginning with John Pearse at Bromsgrove hospital near Birmingham, followed by Neil Dallas at Bristol a year later in which live surgery with CC TV coverage was used to demonstrate IOL and extracapsular advances in surgical technique and new lens designs. These were followed in 1980 with a meeting by Eric Arnott, at Charing Cross Hospital in London in which phacoemulsification techniques were demonstrated by Eric and Bob Sinskey from the US. This was followed in the same year with a meeting by Walter Rich in the Exeter area, and in 1981, by Peter Choyce who organised his meeting at Southend-on-Sea. With the formation of the European Intraocular Implant Council (EIIC) by Cornelius Binkhorst and the first of its conferences at The Hague in 1982, which most of us attended, it was our turn in Ireland to host a conference on implant surgery for UKIOIS.

Controversies in Lens Implant Surgery UKIOIS Killarney 1983:

Ever since Ridley's original lens implant in 1949, controversy has raged regarding the technique of implantation of an artificial lens into the eye during cataract extraction. Most of this originated at Moorfields Eye Hospital in London emanating from Sir Stewart Duke Elder, at the Institute of Ophthalmology and which had continued up to the present in a paper by anterior segment surgeon, Mr. Noel Rice entitled "Why I have reservations about intraocular lens implants".[10] As his concerns and those of others had been primarily directed at lenses implanted in front of the pupil in the anterior chamber extremely close to the cornea or front window of the eye, I particularly concentrated on inviting surgeons from Europe, UK and the US who were using these types of lens implants. The meeting took place at the Europa Hotel overlooking the beautiful lakes of Killarney during the summer of 1983 and was attended by 170 delegates.

Prominent amongst the US delegates was Charles Kelman, Richard Lindstrom, John Alpar, Jerry Freeman, Jack Docick, Jack Kearney, Austen Fink, Dick Keats, and Bob Drews.

Prominent from the UK were Drs. Eric Arnott, John Pearse, Piers Percival, Peter Choyce, Emanuel Rosen, Leonard Luri, Dermot Pierse, Tom Casey, Gordon Catford, and Mr. Ernest Ford (Rayner).

Also present were Christopher Huber (Switzerland), Jan Worst (The Nederlands), José Luis Menezo (Valencia, Spain), Enrico Gallenga and Fabiola Dossi (Italy), Albert Galand (Belgium).

As each surgeon had their own particular lens implant that they were using at the time, extremely animated discussion followed each presentation. Whereas Jan Worst from The Nederlands was advocating his Iris Clip Lobster Claw lens, others such as Kelman

---
10 Rice, N.: "Reservations about IOL'S" – RSM Meeting

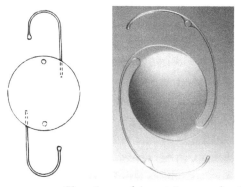
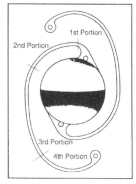

Shearing and Arnott Intraocular Lens Implants

were more in favour of his Quadriflex angle supported lens. Emanuel Rosen reported on his experiences with the Azar angle supported lenses in which degradation of the loop material necessitated their removal. Following two days the meeting concluded with many of the delegates finding time to enjoy the magnificent scenery of Killarney or enjoying a round of golf in Ballybunion.

Lens Implant Cataract Surgery in Ireland – The Beginnings 1976–1988:

The standard cataract operation carried out when I first returned to Waterford in 1973 was the intracapsular operation involving an incision large enough to use a freezing technique to remove the complete lens including its capsule containing the cataract from the eye. Following removal of the cataract, the 12 mm incision was stitched up and the patient was kept in hospital for a day or two to ensure good recovery.

Having attended his courses on intraocular lens implantation and got to know Mr. Peter Choyce from my time in London in 1970, I immediately started to use his Rayner Mark X1 anterior chamber, angle fixated intraocular lens implant in Waterford, which had been approved by the FDA in the US and was being used extensively there. However, bearing in mind Barraquer's original experience in having had to remove many of his anterior chamber lenses implants after intracapsular extraction, and Binkhorst's methodical experiences with different techniques, by 1977, the concept of extracapsular cataract extraction with lens implantation behind the pupil, seem to be finally accepted. From then on, implant technology changed with an emphasis on stabilising the lens in the lens capsule remnants after removal of the cataract itself. Foremost in the UK, Mr. John Pearce from Redditch who had been using the Ridley procedure for some time, started to use his own designed Pearce tripod lens placed in the capsular bag.

From 1977, I continued to use the extracapsular technique with fixation of the lens implant within the capsular bag with excellent results while attending the various conferences at the time. During that period, I used several different types of lens implants depending on the individual conditions in each eye such as the Shearing, Sinskey and Arnott lens implants which produced excellent results. Having acquired considerable amount of experience over a five-year period, I organised a conference in Waterford on Intraocular Lens Implantation over a weekend in May 1982 and invited Prof Robert Drews, President of the International Intraocular Implant Council (IIIC) and small incision Phacoemulsification surgeon, Dr. Donald Prager from the US to join with Dr. Dermot Pierse from the UK and Pharmacia, the manufacturers of the viscoelastic substance, Healon. It was about this time that we started using viscoelastic inside the eye during cataract and corneal transplant surgery to further increase the safety of the operation.[11]

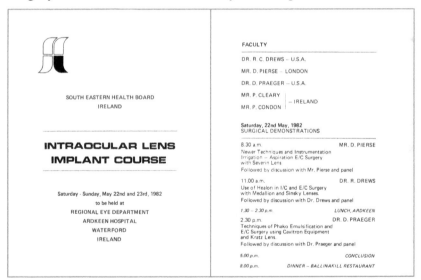

Intraocular Lens Implant Course Waterford 1982

---

11 Condon, P.I., Fitzgerald, G., Burke, A., Gallagher, J.: "The Physical Effects of Visco Elastic Substances on Human Donor Cornea" Trans. Ophthal. Soc. UK Vol.103, 3: 265-267, 1983.

Attendance by consultants at the meeting was extremely encouraging with around 40 representing the major eye hospitals and clinics north and south of the border.

IIIC Membership 1982:

Following our meeting in Waterford, I received a notice shortly afterwards from the secretary of the IIIC, followed by a letter from the chairman, Harold Ridley, indicating that I had been unanimously elected to a membership in the Council at the meeting in San Francisco, an honour which I still retain to this day.

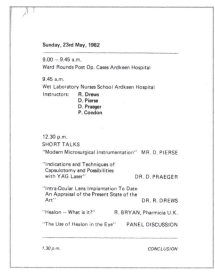

Intraocular Lens Implant Course Waterford 1982

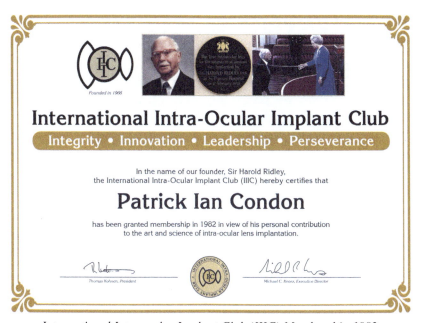

International Intraocular Implant Club (IIIC) Membership 1982

European Intraocular Implant Council (EIIC) 1982:

As the Irish representative on the board of the EIIC, I attended the First EIIC conference in The Hague.

Keyhole Surgery for Cataract:" Phacoemulsification and Foldable Lens Implant Technology 1981:

Phacoemulsification was the term used by Dr. Charles Kelman, at the Manhattan Eye and Ear Hospital, in New York in the early '60s when he discovered that he could use the ultrasound energy of a dental drill to emulsify the inside of the natural lens of the eye. Over a 10-year period, he developed the Cavitron phacoemulsification machine which used a very fine vibrating instrument tip inside the eye augmented by a constant flow of cooled irrigating balanced saline solution surrounding the tip. Whereas the logistics of focusing the energy specifically to the end of the instrument tip through a small 3.2 mm incision, without producing internal heat damage to the eye, presented an enormous challenge to the engineers, the security of the tiny incision facilitated a rapid recovery from the operation with full mobility within days of the surgery. Following intensive research and development into the safety of the technology by Cavitron, the result was a highly sophisticated probe, the titanium tip of which oscillated at 57,000 cycles per second in a longitudinal direction with an excursion of 0.4 mu capable of emulsifying the cataractous material and removing it from the eye with a peristaltic aspiration pump system. Despite the novelty of the idea and its obvious possible advantages, the uptake of phacoemulsification and small incision surgery was delayed considerably by the cost of the Cavitron instrument itself, the cumbersome use of the large hand-piece and the unavailability of suitable foldable intraocular lenses to be able to squeeze through such a small incision. However, with a series of instruction courses, between 1974 and

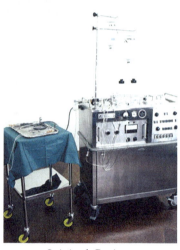

Original Cavitron Phacoemulsification machine

1984, organised in the US by Drs. Kratz, Knolle, Thornton and Kraff, and improved design of the equipment, many more of the younger surgeons who were greatly in favour of ambulatory day care surgical options, began attending Kelman's courses between 1984 and 1988.

It was during this period, that I contacted Dr. Kelman to arrange to visit with him and attend his operating list in New York. Working with Dr. Charles Kelman, known affectionately in the profession as Charlie, turned out to be a novel experience in that the day began at 7 am attending his office in the Empire State

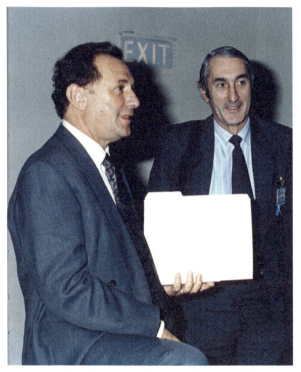

Dr. Charles Kelman and Patrick Condon 1984–88

Building, travelling down to one of the piers on the Hudson River where his helicopter was parked waiting for him to pilot us to the hospital to see the pre-surgical patients. Following the usual checks with air traffic control, we were given clearance to take off. On the way to the hospital, getting a wonderful view of Manhattan as we travelled, our journey involved flying over one of his golf clubs, to find it was covered in snow and that he, alas!, would be unable to play golf later that day.

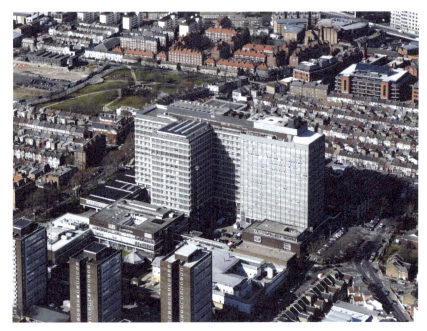

Charing Cross Hospital, Fulham, London Cropped

On arrival at the hospital, his patients were waiting for him in their ordinary clothes, fully prepared by the nurse. Watching him operate using the rather cumbersome phacoemulsification instrumentation through such a small incision with the need to further open the incision to insert a large anterior chamber angle fixated intraocular lens implant, was fascinating. Every movement was highly efficient with no wastage of time between cases. After the operating list was finished, all patients gathered in the waiting area while Charlie talked which each one, checking their operated eyes before we departure from the hospital back to Manhattan

Meanwhile, Eric Arnott, who was now a consultant in Charing Cross Hospital London and a great friend of Charles Kelman, had already started using the original Cavitron instrument in 1979, and had begun to organise courses and demonstrations with live surgery in London. Having worked with him as a junior doctor at the Royal Eye Hospital, he asked me to assist him in surgery during several courses with American surgeons in London. This was when I first met with Richard Packard, his senior registrar at the time. During these visits to London usually at weekend courses organised by Eric, I learned a lot from Cavitron in how to set up wet laboratory facilities for surgeons to learn the extra skills required for small incision surgery and the logistics of bringing this technology into the operating theatre environment.

In 1984, the FDA approved the use of the foldable Mazzocco hydrophobic silicone lens implant for use in the US. Almost coincidentally, polymer scientists were beginning to develop softer plastic materials with refractive ability which could be used in the manufacturing of optical lenses capable of being folded and inserted into the eye through small incisions. One of these was a Dr. Graham Barrett, an ophthalmic surgeon at the Lions Institute in Perth, Western Australia, who had developed a hydrophilic acrylic polyHema 38% water content autoclavable, biocompatible soft intraocular lens implant that could also be inserted through a smaller 6 mm incision. With the purchase of the product licence by Alcon Laboratories, at Fort Worth, Texas, US, the IOGEL intraocular lens implant was subjected to the usual investigations

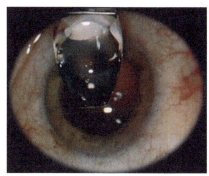

Foldable Hydrogel Intraocular single piece lens Implant

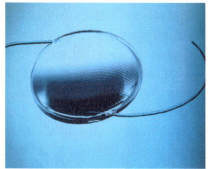

Foldable Hydrogel intraocular 3-piece lens implant

Hydrogel Intraocular Lens Experience With Endocapsular Implantation

W. J. RICH,[1] P. I. CONDON,[2] S. P. B. PERCIVAL[3]

Exeter, Waterford, Scarborough.

Summary

The experience is presented of three independent surgeons using Hydrogel posterior chamber intraocular lenses in a combined series of 157 endocapsular cataract extractions. One hundred and fifty of these eyes were examined after a minimum follow–up period of one year and 92.0% achieved visual acuity of 6/12 or better, and 98.6% achieved this if pre-existing pathology was excluded. Insertion of this lens has proved to be simple, the adaptions of technique required are described and the complications are presented and analysed.

Hydrogel Intraocular Lens Experience with Endocapsular Implantation.

and scrutiny required by the FDA and approval by them for use within Europe. Not having the facilities for phacoemulsification in the UK or Ireland at the time, and in conjunction with Drs. Walter Rich, in Exeter and Piers Percival in Harrogate, and myself in Waterford, we began to insert the unfolded IOGEL lens through a 6 mm incision.[12]

US Influence and Irish Cataract and Lens Implant Surgery 1983-88:

With the realisation that much of the stimulus for further development in cataract surgery was happening in the US, I started to attend the American Society of Contemporary Ophthalmology meetings which were usually held in Florida at a time when discussions on the development of the US Ambulatory Day Care Centres for Cataract Surgery was ongoing. The introduction and acceptance by cataract surgeons in the US of phacoemulsification and small incision surgery with the reduced need for hospitalisation, had prompted US surgeons to question the Government's remuneration system for hospitals. It was at these meetings, that I first met with Dr. John R. Kearney, generally known as Jack, an ophthalmic surgeon from Gloversville, Upstate New York, who had qualified in medicine in Dublin at the Royal College of Surgeons, and who was very familiar with Ireland. As a fully committed small incision phacoemulsification cataract surgeon and involved a lot with the manufacturing companies in the design of intraocular lens implants and surgical instrumentation, I learned a lot about how we should make progress in Ireland. While attending these meetings on an annual basis and travelling to visit some of the doctors' clinics to observe the logistical organisation of their practices, I soon felt that there was a lot to be learned from the practice of ophthalmology and cataract surgery in the US. As a result, a group of US-based ophthalmologists decided in 1982 to form the Irish American Ophthalmological Society with U.S.-based, Dr. John Kearney and myself on the Irish side, the object being to increase ophthalmological links between ophthalmologists on both sides of the Atlantic.

---

12 Rich, W. J., Condon, P.I., Percival S.P: "Hydrogen Intraocular Lens Experience with Endo capsular Implantation", Eye 2, 5232-528. 1988.

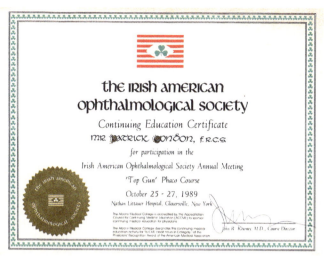

Irish American Ophthalmological Society Membership

This organisation which catalysed a major transfer of information to Irish ophthalmologists, proved to be extremely beneficial in encouraging relationships between the two transatlantic groups, An example of this, was the visit by a group of us from the north and south of Ireland to the Gimbal Institute at Calgary, Ontario, Canada in October 1989, on our way to the American Academy of Ophthalmology annual meeting in the US. Dr Gimbal himself was known to be the first person with Prof Thomas Neuhann, in Munich, Germany, to develop the technique of capsulorhexis or capsular tearing of the lens capsule prior to removal of the cataract. His clinic had the reputation of being organised in a most efficient manner, utilising ambulatory day care cataract surgery, which was becoming the norm in the US. He also introduced us to the use of topical anaesthesia with preoperative decompression of the eye. The group then journeyed on to the Boston area where the Irish American Ophthalmological Society hosted the "Top Gun Phaco Meeting" attended by Charlie Kelman and Michael Blumenthal from Israel who arrived by helicopter.

One of the developments which was interesting to observe, was the technological advance in phacoemulsification ultrasound instrumentation. With Cavitron upgrading their handpiece probe technology, other companies such as Storz, Chiron and Allergan came up with alternative types of aspiration pump systems, some of which were more efficient than others at maintaining anterior chamber depth during surgery. One of these was by a company called Optical Microsurgical Systems designed by Dr. Jim Little, which had a very sophisticated digital irrigation aspiration pump system with a light flexible handpiece.

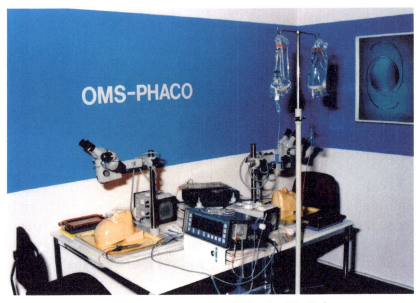

Optical Micro Surgical Phacoemulsification Wet Laboratory

With the establishment of the European OMS agency in Belgium by the late, Guy Van de Weyer, in the mid-80s, I approached the company with a view to setting up a small wet laboratory in Waterford for ophthalmologists to come and practice learning the technique of using this equipment. While many surgeons in Ireland were extremely competent at using the standard extracapsular technique, the use of phacoemulsification with a vibrating probe inside the eye, involved quite a different technique demanding considerable skill. Anxious to establish a footprint in Ireland, an OMS Diplomat machine, was lent to us by the company which we used with pigs' eyes retrieved from the abattoir to practice on in the wet lab. After some experience in the laboratory, we then began to use phacoemulsification for adult cataracts using a 3.25 mm corneal incision. By the mid-80s, I started to use the technique for most cataracts, developing a folding forceps for the Barrett IOGEL lens, injecting it through the 3.25 mm incision. By 1988, I had carried out 150 successful phacoemulsification procedures.

Following the almost simultaneous reporting of the technique of capsulorhexis by Thomas Neuhann in Germany and Howard Gimbel in Canada, I immediately started developing the skills required to accomplish it and bought a Utrata forceps for this purpose, which instrument maker John Weiss subsequently modified for me (Condon Capsulorhexis Forceps).

1st Conference Ireland: "Phacoemulsification and Small Incisions" – Waterford Regional 1988.

Building on a good relationship with OMS, I decided to invite Dr. Bill Maloney from San Diego, Calif. rand Prof. Richard Keats, Prof. of Ophthalmology at Ohio State University, Columbus, Ohio, US, Dr. Graham Wright, Rochdale, UK and Dr. Charles Cory, Redhill, UK, all of whom were practising phacoemulsification surgeons to come to the Waterford Regional Eye department in September 1988 for the first all-Ireland conference on "Phacoemulsification and Small Incision Surgery for Cataracts". Dr. Maloney, an expert in phacoemulsification in the US, spoke on his "3-Step Phacoemulsification Technique" followed by a second presentation on the "Management of Residual Astigmatism", while Prof Keats spoke on the "The Value of Phaco Course Education" for surgeons beginning phacoemulsification surgery. I demonstrated a phacoemulsification procedure and outlined some of the techniques that helped me initially. The course was attended by Mr. Philip Cleary, Mr. Eamon Horan and Mr. Aidan Murray, (Cork Regional), Mr. Brendan Young, (Limerick Regional), Mr. Peter Barry (St. Vincent's Hospital, and Mr Frank Lavery, (Dublin), Mr. Patrick Johnston, Mr. Stuart Johnston, Mr. Gerry Kervick and Mr. P. Redmond, (Belfast), Mr. Patrick Hayes, Peter Tormey and me, (Waterford Regional). Others attending were Dr. Joe Eustace, Dr. Shay Ford, Dr. Louis Ryan, Dr. Margaret Pierse, Mr. Jim Lavin, Mr. David Leighton from the UK and Mr. Everard Hewson (Galway University Hospital).

By the end of 1989, with its technical and surgical achievements, the unit at Waterford Regional Hospital had introduced a successful ambulatory day care surgery admission system with the ability for patients to be reviewed by the operating surgeon on the day after surgery before being discharged. In September 1992, Dr. Charlie Kelman received the *"National Medal of Technology"* award from President George Bush at the White House for his unique originality and perseverance in the development of phacoemulsification.

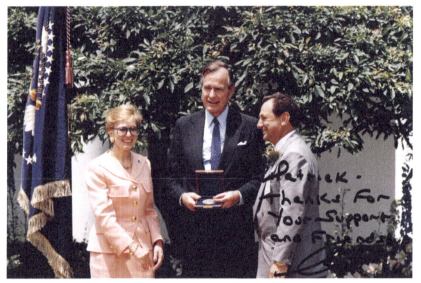

National Medal of Technology Award to Charles Kelman, 1992

UKIOIS – UKISCRS Presidency 1994–1996:

In 1994, I was invited to be President of the United Kingdom Society of Implant and Cataract Surgeons (UKICS), one of my objectives being to re-boot the finances of the society, which we achieved with the help of the ophthalmic oriented companies and support from the members. A decision was also made by Council to change the name of the society to include refractive surgery and Ireland as a country in the name of the society with the rebranding to United Kingdom and Ireland Society of Cataract and Refractive Surgeons (UKISCRS).

UKISCRS 25th Anniversary of Phaco in Europe – 1997:

Since Charles Kelman first spoke on phaco at the OSUK meeting in 1970, Eric Arnott subsequently performed the first phaco in Europe on the 26th October, 1971, followed two years later by Ulrich Dardenne in Germany. They were amongst the

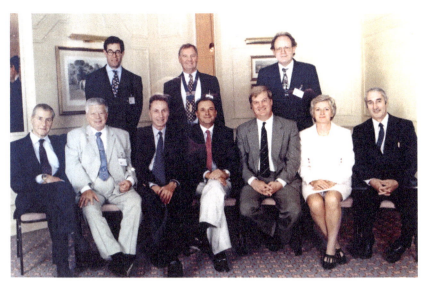

UKISCRS 25th Anniversary of Phaco in Europe 1997

world's first faculty who were still practising, promoting and teaching the technique to present and future international colleagues. On the 18th September, 1997, at the UKISCRS annual meeting in Chester, a symposium to commemorate the 25th Anniversary of Phaco in Europe was held. Faculty members included Charles Kelman USA (Chairman), Eric Arnott UK, (Secretary), Slav Fyodorov (USSR), Hans Reinhardt Koch (Germany), David Apple (USA), James Hunter (UK), Patrick Condon (Ireland), Helen Seward (UK), Robert Sinskey (USA), Richard Packard UK), and Ulrich Dardenne (Germany).

Chapter 13
Blindness from Corneal Disease in UK and Ireland

The cornea is the front window of the eye through which all light and images of objects in the outside world are transmitted to the retina at the back of the eye, from where the images are sent to the brain. The cornea is therefore essential to the provision of sight and when damaged by infection, diseases, or trauma, it can result in significant degrees of impaired vision. Some patients have opaque scarred corneas from long-standing chemical injuries and chronic viral or bacterial infections, while others suffer from extremely thinned corneas due to advanced keratoconus.

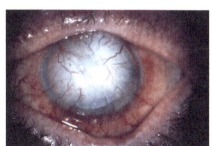

Corneal Blindness – Chemical Injury with severe corneal scarring

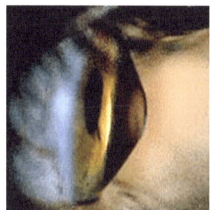

Keratoconus

History of Corneal Transplantation:

The first successful corneal transplant reported in the Dublin Journal of Medical Science, was performed by an Irish ophthalmic surgeon, Dr. Samuel Bigger in 1835. Bigger described performing a corneal allograft transplant in a blind gazelle which he had encountered while being held captive by a nomadic tribe on the outskirts of Cairo. In 1905, Dr. Eduard Zirm, in Austria performed the first corneal transplant on a farmer blind in both eyes from severe lime burns. The donated corneas came from an 11-year-old boy who was blinded in one eye with an embedded intraocular piece of steel, but which had left his cornea perfectly clear and suitable to be donated. In the absence of modern type surgical instruments, the only way in which the damaged cornea could be removed was with a circular 5 mm diameter von Hippel trephine similar in principle to an apple corer.

Following a very successful result with full restoration of his sight in the eye, the second eye was operated in a similar way using a deceased organ donor cornea. While it was commonly known at the time that solid organs in the body from a donor were prone to rejection by the recipient's body because of immune incompatibility, the reason put forward for the success of transplanting the cornea from one individual to another without the need for tissue typing and cross matching, was the lack of blood vessels in the cornea, which isolates it from the immune system of the rest of the body, making it an immunologically privileged area. Following a succession of similar cases and with continuing research and evolving technology, Zirm established his eye bank in rural Austria, which subsequently treated 47,000 patients. In 1944, Dr. R. Townley Paton started to carry out corneal transplant procedures at the Manhattan Eye Ear and Throat Hospital in New York and founded the world's first eye bank, the Eye Bank for Sight Restoration in New York. By 1957, there were 12 eye banks in the United States, all of which united in 1961 to form the Eye Banks Association of America (EBAA)

Cornea – Plastic and Eye Bank Unit, Queen Victoria Hospital, East Grinstead:

In 1945, Sir Benjamin Rycroft, OBE, FRCS, a post-war veteran ophthalmic surgeon and consultant at Moorfields and several general hospitals in south London, was approached by Sir Archibald McIndoe, famous for his successful surgery on mutilated and burned pilots at the Queen Victoria Hospital in East Grinstead, to establish an eye department within the unit. With the birth of the Cornea -Plastic Unit in East Grinstead, Rycroft gathered momentum in his work. With an outstanding contribution to lacrimal, eyelid, orbital surgery and particularly ptosis, he also specialised in corneal transplant work. In 1952, he was responsible for initiating a national campaign for a corneal grafting act. The campaign which was supported by the Royal College of Surgeons and the South-East Regional Hospital Board, was passed in 1952 and with it the first United Kingdom Eye Bank was established in East Grinstead. The act was later passed in 1961 and broadened to include other human tissue and is now known as the Human Tissue Act.

In 1967, Mr. Thomas Aquinas Casey, FRCS, a graduate from University College Dublin, consultant ophthalmologist at the Westminster and Middlesex hospitals, was appointed as Medical Director to the Cornea – Plastic Unit, extending Sir Benjamin's role as a corneal surgeon and taking over the organisation of the Eye Bank. During his tenure at East Grinstead, Mr. Casey published widely which is encapsulated in his book entitled "Corneal Grafting: Principles and Practice" by Casey, T. A. and Mayer, D.J., which was published in 1984.

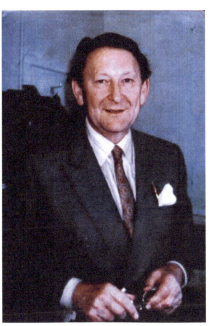

Mr. Thomas Aquinas Casey (1929–1993)

In 1986, with the establishment of the Corneal Transplant Service Eye Bank (CTS) in Bristol, the eye bank services at East Grinstead were gradually phased out. The activities of the unit continued with Mr. Abbe Werb, in oculoplastics and lacrimal surgery and Tom Casey in corneal transplantation until his death in 1992.

Mr. Sheraz Daya, MD, FRCS, FACS, was a graduate from RCS (Dublin), with the experience of working as a Fellow at the University of Minnesota, (US) with Drs. Richard Lindstrom and Edward Holland. After working as Head of Cornea with Dr. David Paton, founder of Orbis, in New York City for several years, he was appointed Director of the unit at East Grinstead in

1993. For 8 years he continued with the development of corneal transplantation and oculoplastic extending into refractive surgery until his retirement from the NHS in 2011. Following his move to private practice at the purpose-built Centre for Sight clinic in East Grinstead, his practice has advanced into the more special aspects of corneal and cataract treatments.

International Refractive Update Conference – Mater Hospital 2nd Dec. 2005.
The Thomas Aquinas Casey Memorial Lecturer

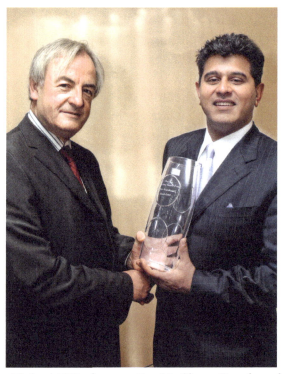

Professor Michael O'Keefe presenting Mr. Sheraz Dayah on delivering the Thomas Aquinas Casey Memorial Lecture 2005

Eye Donation and UK Corneal Transplant Service Eye Bank (CTS):

Whereas live donations occur with donation of a kidney from a healthy person to another person in renal failure, most organ donation takes place after death and until recently required permission from next of kin. Deceased organ donation now exists all over the world and in the UK and Ireland the Corneal Transplant Service Eye Bank (CTS) depends on the carrying a donor card which authenticates the donor's permission for the donation. This allows for rapid recovery of the donated eyes after death. There is also the situation where an untimely death can occur either by accident or in hospital, in which case consent from the next of kin would be required.

With the opening of the new surgical eye operating theatre in 1976, I decided to set up a system of eye donation for relatives of deceased patients at first in Waterford Regional and subsequently extending it to the five general hospitals in the SEAHB area. With the help of the Irish Kidney Association in Beaumont Hospital, Dublin, who were actively retrieving donated kidneys and heart organs from donors in the country, it was not difficult to introduce the idea of eye donation to the hospital management and the public in Waterford at the time. As consent from the relatives of the deceased had always been regarded as a sensitive issue, and as the medical person responsible for recovering the eyes after death, an approach was made to the religious order of nursing professionals on duty at the hospital, to assist with interviewing the relatives about possible donation. With their agreement, I would then be called to recover the eyes in the mortuary. On removal of the donated eyes, hand-painted artificial shells were inserted in their place and the eye lids gently closed with fines stitches. The eyes were then taken to a small refrigerator in the eye theatre sterilising area and kept at -6° C with an antibiotic until the operation was carried out, usually within six hours. With this system, all corneal transplant patients had to be admitted at short notice which involved at times working at night and at unsocial hours. While this local service worked extremely well for several years, we finally began to use the newly developed UK Corneal Transplant Service Eye Bank (CTS) from Bristol which opened in March 1986, and which introduced the technique of organ cultured storage of donated material at 34 degrees Centigrade. The advantages of this method were the extended storage time allowing for more flexibility in transportation of the donated material and the scheduling of surgery for the hospital and patient.

Corneal Transplantation in Ireland – The Beginnings. 1976:

Arriving in Waterford in 1973, I soon encountered patients with advanced corneal diseases requiring full-thickness corneal transplants to restore their sight. Unfortunately, facilities for full-thickness penetrating corneal transplantation were unavailable locally, necessitating referrals elsewhere. To my knowledge, the only places where this could be done successfully were at; the Cornea - Plastic Unit and Eye Bank (UK) in East Grinstead, or Moorfields Hospital, London. With the acquisition of the surgical and Zeiss ceiling mounted operating microscope facilities in the newly built eye unit in 1976, and the possibility of a supply of donor material from the newly opened CTS Eye Bank in Bristol (UK) in 1986, I finally decided to operate on some of the patients with more advanced corneal pathology in Waterford.

My next priority was the acquisition of a suitable trephine system for removal of the diseased portion of the patient's cornea replacing it with a clear donor piece the same size and shape. With a variety of different systems available, the system I chose was the Guided Trephine System invented by Dr. Jorg Krumeich in Bochum, Germany, and used extensively by Professor Thomas Neuhann in Munich and Dr. Sharrer in Frankfurt. It appeared to be the most precise instrument available. The advantage of this trephine system over the others was its ability to flatten the abnormal

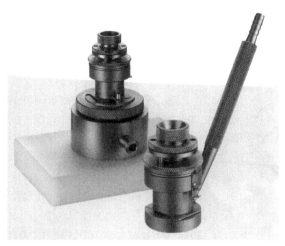

Krumeich Guided Trephine System (GTS)

shape of heavily distorted corneal surfaces with stabilisation of the cutting process during the trephination procedure. The result of this is a complete vertical cut through the centre of the cornea with more accuracy in the replacement and suturing of the donor piece and much less post-operative astigmatism. I was now able to begin an active corneal transplantation service and began receiving patients from eye centres throughout the country.

As the service developed, we began to attract some extremely complicated patients for transplantation and at one stage were regularly doing a graft each week many of whom were young healthy adults who were severely visually handicapped with advanced keratoconus and unable to wear glasses or contact lenses. One patient was a senior government minister from north Dublin, active in politics and coming up for re-election, who had a badly scarred and active viral resistant infection of his cornea. Following a very successful graft procedure with material donated from a deceased donor in the southeast area and a short postoperative recovery period, he subsequently resumed his career and was re-elected.

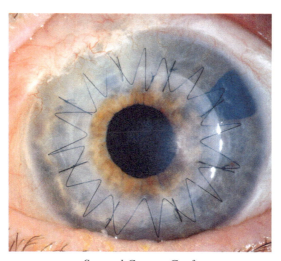

Sutured Cornea Graft

With the increasing development and integration of the regional hospital services throughout the country and the need to quantify the consultant requirements, Comhairle na nOspideal was set up by the Department of Health. With the dramatic development of the ophthalmic services in the SEAHB, I was approached by the DOH offering me a position that would allow me to attend meetings. After a 2-year commitment, Comhairle produced a document entitled "Hospital Ophthalmic Services -A Discussion Document" in which the possibility of an amalgamation of the stand-alone Royal Victoria Eye and Ear Hospital with St. Vincent's Hospital was considered but deemed to be unacceptable by the Sisters of Charity and the board of the hospital subsequently.[13]

---

13 Comhairle na n Ospedale Hospital: "Ophthalmic Services. A Discussion Document"1985-88.

Chapter 14
Eye Trauma – A Serious Problem

The increased incidence of severe eye injuries arriving in casualty at the Regional Eye Unit and other Irish hospitals, began to raise general concern as the services developed. On analysing the source of these injuries, we began to recognise that there was a complete lack of eye protection at every level around the country concerning agriculture, industry, and sport. On examining the facilities in other countries for eye protection in these various activities, we realised that in Ireland, we had been extremely negligent in the provision of eye protection in all aspects of working life and that little if nothing had been done to rectify the situation. In the United States, all industrial unions and sporting organisations had strict rules about the wearing of face and eye protection which was mandatory while engaged at work and involved in sporting activities.

Road Blindness:

When a head-on collision occurs at moderate speed, the motorist (if unrestrained) flexes forwards; the legs press against the floor; the knees strike the dashboard, and the head hits the windscreen. What happens next depends on the composition of the glass. On impact the monolithic toughened glass windscreen, in common use in the UK and Ireland at the time, may shatter into multiple polygonal fragments. This offers little resistance to the head, which ploughs through the windscreen all the way to the lower framework with serious risks of lacerations to the face and eyes. When the eyes are damaged, the typical injuries are cornea scleral perforation, prolapse of the iris or pupil, and opacification or dislocation of the lens from the eye. Even with modern microsurgical techniques, the internal damage is often so severe that many of these eyes are permanently blinded or may even have to be enucleted or removed. When the motorist is wearing a safety belt, the risk to the eyes from windscreens, though greatly reduced, is not eliminated. In a collision, the body cannot move forwards, but the impact can still cause a toughened windscreen to shatter and then disintegrate. The windscreen may also be broken by direct external forces such as a stone or animal so that 15 to 20 lb. of compressed glass explodes into the vehicle. In the case of laminated windscreens, a crack in a web like fashion occurs but generally the windscreen remaining intact.

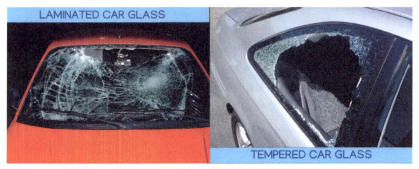

Windscreen Glass. Tempered -vs- Laminated

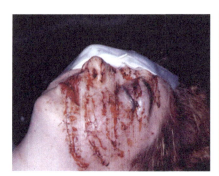

Severe Windscreen Facial and Eye Injuries

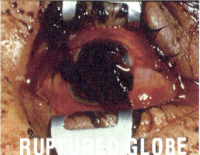

Severe Windscreen Facial and Eye Injuries. Ruptured Globe

Seat Belt Regulation Changes:

The introduction by the Road Traffic Act in Feb 1971, of a law which made it mandatory to wear seat belts in all vehicles, reduced significantly the number of accidents to the eyes and face of those involved in car accidents. However, it had little effect on those injuries sustained from shattered glass of the older toughened windscreens.

Drink Driving Law Changes:

In June, 1974, the alcohol limit for driving a car was reduced which in the absence of of any changes in laminated windscreen legislation, made very little difference to the accident rate. As a result, hospital casualty departments were still being kept busy.

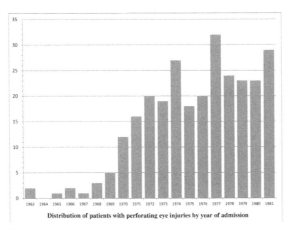

Graphic Increase in Incidence of Windscreen Injuries

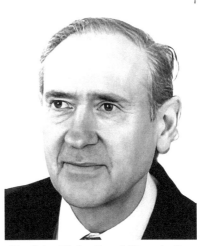

Mr. John Blake, Royal Victoria Eye and Ear Hospital, Dublin

Following realisation by the American Academy of Ophthalmology of the benefit of inserting laminated windscreens in motor cars for the prevention of severe eye injuries involved in motor accidents in the US, legislated was introduced in 1966 mandating that laminated windscreens be fitted to all motor vehicles. In Ireland, it was Drs. John Blake and Geraldine Kelly at St. Vincent's Hospital, Dublin, that brought to our attention the serious rise in severe eye injuries from such accidents, reporting statistics of eye injuries in a major publication in 1983 and subsequently in a letter in the British Medical Journal on "Road Blindness".[14] Based on this evidence,

---

14 Blake, J. "Road Blindness", Brit. Medical Jour. Vol.287, 626-627, 3rd Sept. 1983.

successful lobbying of the government to introduce mandatory laminated windscreens in all new cars in Ireland, was eventually introduced in 1986.

Industrial Injuries:

The National Irish Safety Organisation (NISO) was originally set up by the Government in 1963 and was used to bolster the Factories Act of 1955 and the Factories Advisory Council to reduce the increasing numbers of industrial accidents at the time. Throughout the '70s, NISO opened its doors to individual members as well as organisations, who could join to study and promote health and safety. In the '80s, NISO contributed to the development of the Safety Industry Act which amended the Factories Act of 1955. This improved working conditions by adding the obligation on employers to provide and implement an added safety statement and make more precise the functional role of safety representatives and committees.

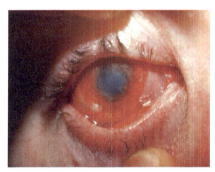

Severe acute corneal, conjunctival and eyelid chemical burs

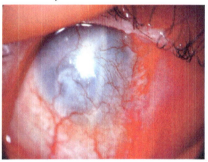

Chronic scarring of the cornea with conjunctival adhesions

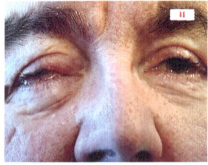

Chemical eye burns with complete blindness in one and partial sight in the other

By 1989, the Safety, Health and Welfare at Work Act was passed. This led to the creation of the Health and Safety Authority. Despite all the legislated measures being slowly put into place and the work of safety organisations, such as NISO and others, severe eye and head accidents continued to flow into our eye casualty units throughout the country. In the case of the safety organisations and large industries, this was being covered by in-house talks and lectures on general safety by members of the medical profession in which eyecare was included. However, where the public was concerned or those not associated with a safety organisation, such as pertained in a large factory institution, or in a situation on their own in a small business, there was very little incentive to be conscious about the need for eye safety measures. In addition to this, the malaise of the public in general against the wearing of seatbelts and attitude to drink driving, with delays by the government to legislate on the issue of laminated windscreens, did little to reduce this degree of trauma.

Agricultural Injuries:

Farmers and agricultural workers on the land, often working independently on their own with large agricultural machinery in all sorts of varying weather conditions, can often be faced with sudden mechanical problems that need immediate fixing. As well as having to deal with toxic chemicals, repairing machinery, the use of welding equipment, and repairing tractor equipment, farmers are constantly being exposed to eye injury prone situations. The use of chain saws without adequate head and face protection can have serious consequences. One injury, particularly common in the farming community, is the penetration into the eye of a steel splinter while hammering a metal object which requires its removal with complicated vitreoretinal surgery

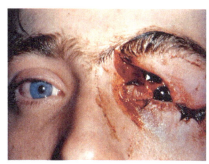

Blunt trauma – Chainsaw laceration of eye lid and total loss of eye

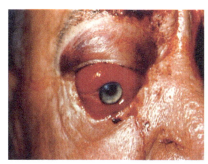

Massive orbital and periorbital haemorrhage from severe eye trauma

Sport Injuries – Hurling Squash and Badminton:

The story of Tom Walsh from Thomastown, Co Kilkenny, highlights the severe eye injury that might result from sport. Tom was a member of the introductory team from 1963-67 and was the captain of the Kilkenny side in the 1967 All Ireland final against Tipperary in Croke Park. Kilkenny won the game but in the closing stages of the contest, Tom was struck by a blow to the head by an opposition hurley and fell to the ground with blood pouring from his left eye. He was subsequently rushed to the Royal Victoria Eye and Ear Hospital in Dublin, where he underwent surgery to remove what was left of the damaged eye. While Tipperary had dominated over Kilkenny since 1922, Kilkenny went on to win the match. Tom recovered from the injury, but lost all sight in his left eye, which put a permanent end to his sporting career.

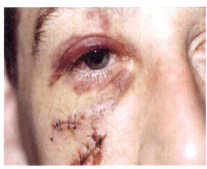

Laceration of face and cheek bone area from hurling injury

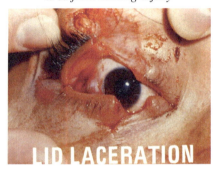

Total laceration of eye lids and damage to the eye from hurling

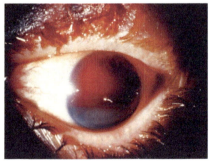

Internal haemorrhage of the eye from a direct blow from a hurley

Some time after this incident happened in 1967, another young man in his early twenties was admitted under my care after a similar accident occurred while he was engaged in a practice session with a local Waterford team. It seemed that a hurley from a nearby player slipped from his grip making a direct hit on this young boys right eye. Unfortunately, due to the fact that the eye was completely damaged beyond repair and could possibly affect the good eye with a condition called sympathetic ophthalmitis, the remains of the damaged eye had to be surgically removed. In reviewing the nature of the accident subsequently, it transpired that no helmets or eye protection had been worn during the practice session.

Because of the smaller size of the ball in squash and the shuttlecock in badminton, injuries caused in these sports usually result in a blunt type concussion injury to the eye with internal bleeding and retinal damage, rather than perforation.

Gardening Accidents:

Chopping sticks, hammering nails, strimming lawns, and using wire brushes and rakes are all garden activities which can cause very severe eye injuries and are preventable with the proper eye protection.

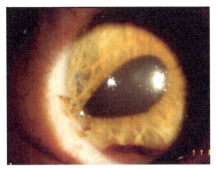

Perforation of the eyeball from a stone while strimming

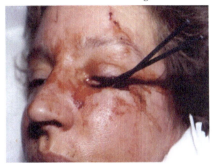

Pieces of a garden rake penetrating the eye

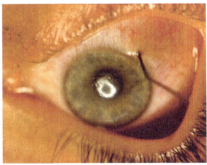

Pieces of a wire brush penetrating the eye

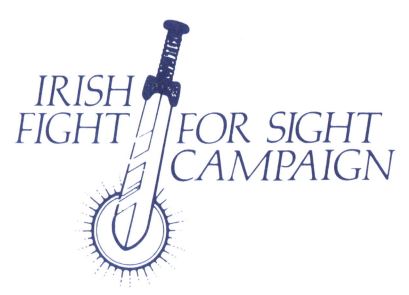

Irish Fight for Sight Logo

Chapter 15
Prevention of Blindness Programmes 1984

The Fight for Sight Concept – And Those that Made It Happen

Based on the experiences of severe eye trauma encountered at Waterford Regional Eye department and other hospitals throughout the country from 1973 to 1984, an average of 25,000 cases were estimated to occur per year in Ireland. It was therefore logical to assume the need for a more active approach to the public with information on the use of eye protection in certain working conditions and sporting activities.

Having spoken to a great many international organisations regarding eye protection programs in other countries, especially in the US, it seemed that approaching people directly in their own sphere of work or sporting activity, was the only way in which this could be achieved with any degree of success. Whereas ophthalmologists are those that see at first hand, the devastating and tragic effects of major eye injury, it was felt that the only way that this could be changed, was for concerned members of the of the community to become involved in a public awareness programme supported by prominent leaders of business and major health organisations. As a result, a charitable organisation called Irish Fight for Sight Campaign was set up

Foundation of Irish Fight for Sight Campaign Objective: June 1984.

1. To increase public awareness of the value of sight and to actively advocate the use of eye protection devices for those participating in sport, agriculture, industry and engineering activities.

2. To donate diagnostic and therapeutic equipment to eye units in Irish hospitals.
3. To fund scientific research into the origins, nature and treatment of eye diseases in Ireland.
4. To initiate prevention of blindness programs relative to cataract, glaucoma, corneal and diabetic eye disease.

On 19th September 1984, at the inaugural meeting of the Irish Fight for Sight Campaign, the constitution of the organisation as a charitable body was ratified and Mr. Bobby Kerr, hotel proprietor and developer of the Kilkenny-based New Park hotel, was appointed chairman of the meeting. The other founding members were Mr. James Kennedy, Managing Director, of the European headquarters of Bausch & Lomb – Manufacturer of Contact Lenses in Waterford – and myself as consultant ophthalmic surgeon to the SEAHB.

The meeting opened with my report outlining the eye trauma experience at Waterford Regional Eye department over the 10-year period between 1973 and 1984 and the report by doctors John Blake and Geraldine Kelly from St. Vincent's Hospital, on the devastating effect produced by toughened windscreens in cars in road traffic accidents in Ireland. The discussion broadened to include some of the severe chemical injuries produced by acids and alkalis and the severe injuries sustained by hurlers in the GAA. Having accepted my report with the obvious need for the setting up of an active accident prevention programme, various methods for tackling the situation were discussed:

1. Increased promotion of eye safety programs in factories, engineering businesses, agriculture and official government organisations.
2. Increased communication of eye safety to the public.
3. The lobbying of politicians and civil servants with a view to promoting the concept of eye protection through legislation and politics.
4. Tackling the GAA's entrenched resistance to the wearing of eye protection in the sport of hurling.

Following the initial discussion on the formidable task ahead for the IFFS, it was agreed that Mrs. June Darrer, hotel proprietor

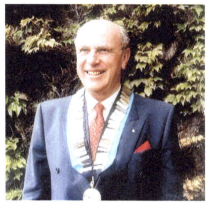

Mr. Bobby Kerr, New Park Hotel, Kilkenny

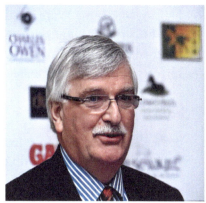

Mr. James Kennedy, Managing Director of Bausch and Lomb, Contact Lens Mfd. Co. Waterford

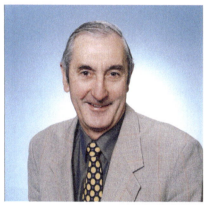

Mr. Patrick Condon, Consultant Ophthalmic Surgeon, SEAHB

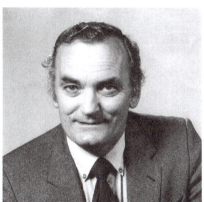

Mr. Jim McGrath, McGrath Opticians and Sefton Optical, Waterford

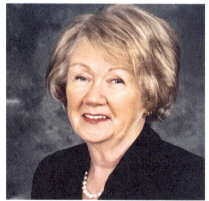

Mrs. June Darrer, Dooley's Hotel, Waterford

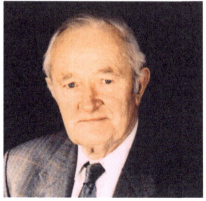

Mr. Michael Collins Managing Director Clover Meats

of Dooley's Hotel, Waterford, proposed by Bobby Kerr, Mr. Michael Collins, Managing Director of Clover Meets, Ferrybank, Waterford, and Mr. James P. McGrath, McGrath Opticians, Waterford, proposed by me, should be asked to join the board.

Primary Issues for the IFFS Board

1. Awareness of Eye Protection: It was agreed that I would be personally responsible for this aspect of the campaign by giving slideshow presentations to groups of workers and members of the public on our 10-year report of eye injuries and the need for protection. It was also hoped that the goodwill generated by the successful care given to individual patients at the hospital in Waterford, would lay the grounds for the formation of eye safety committees in the localities from which they came and that would both stimulate and finance the continued promotion of eye safety in the areas.
2. Financial Support: The generation of adequate finances to run such a campaign would require employment of a full-time executive officer and an office.

Irish Fight for Sight Campaign (IFFS) – Initial Issues

Patrons:

The first patron of IFFS was Dr. Patrick Hillary, President of Ireland from 1976 to 1990, followed by Dr. Mary Robinson, President from 1990 to 1997, followed by Mary McAleese from 1997 to 2011, followed by Michael D. Higgins from 2011 to 2017.

Much discussion centred around the design of a suitable logo for IFFS, based on the concept of a Sword of Light conjuring up hope for those in darkness due to eye problems. It was decided that surrounding the image of the sword, "Irish Fight" would be placed on one side and "For Sight Campaign" on the other side, with an image of the eye with the sun's rays emanating from the tip of the sword.

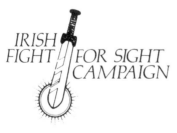

Irish Fight for Sight Logo

Office /Development Officer:

Office accommodation was eventually provided at number 4, Parnell St. Waterford and a Mr. Mike Garvey was appointed as Development Officer with a degree of executive function. His contract involved the organising and attendance at meetings organised by committee members at venues throughout the country, generating finances for the campaign and offering support to members of the public interested in joining the campaign. His salary would come from the monies generated through the campaign.

Accountant:

Mr. Kevin Hall, of accountancy firm of Hall Lifford Hall, was appointed accountant.

IFFS Local Meetings:

Notices were placed in the local newspaper in each county with information about IFFS, pointing out its charitable status and the four objectives of the campaign, the main one of which was to bring to the public a greater awareness of the need to wear eye protection when necessary. Public meetings were generally held in local hotels at which I would speak about eye protection in various occupations and the services being developed by the SEAHB at the Waterford Regional Hospital. Invitations would also be sent out to the local general practitioners, nursing professionals, community care workers and members of the National Council for the Blind, all of whom became both interested and supportive in what we were doing. Invariably, people with eye problems and especially those who had received treatment at Waterford would show up for the meeting, many of whom would have questions about themselves or their relatives.

After some months, it soon became obvious that we needed to have a proper information brochure and video material available with our logo, office address and phone number so that people could communicate with the office. Furthermore, it was decided to print a IFFS Campaign Newsletter four times a year with up-to-date information about the campaign and its activities.

Formation of IFFS Committees:
Industrial and Educational:

The first committee to be formed by IFFS was the Industrial and Educational committee. Chaired by John Condon, Managing Director of Merck Sharpe & Dohme (Clonmel), members included Safety officers Ms Assumpta O'Mahony (MSD), Ann Marie Fogarty (Bausch and Lomb), Ms Maidie Carroll (Waterford Crystal), Maurice Dougan, Optician (Clonmel), Vincent Gallagher (PPI Adhesives, Waterford), and Tom McDermot, (Digital, Ireland), which represented a good cross-section of some of the major companies in the south-east. The aim of this committee was to bring high safety issues into the workplace of all industries in the area.

A Corporate Membership Scheme was set up to allow companies to receive all information material from IFFS. This included:

1. Free admission to IFFS seminars and meetings including those on special industrial and education topics.
2. The availability of speakers to address the company's board or employees.
3. Free access to all education and information materials including videos, films, newsletters, posters etcetera.
4. Practical advice and support in setting up an in-house eye safety program in the company's workplace, school, community hall, sports club or whatever.
5. Advice to companies in arranging meetings for the workers in the organisation to help raise awareness of the risk to sight and the preservation measures to counteract the risks.

Companies were also expected to ensure that all workers were made aware of the dangers to their sight in high-risk situations by wearing protective eye wear and the posting of signs and display posters on eye protection. In return, IFFS would also appreciate any ideas the company and its workers might have as regards fundraising for charity.

While this committee was approaching several of the larger firms in the south-east through semi-state general safety organisations such as NISO, a considerable number of companies involved in very high-risk activities without any safety cover were discovered. These included small engineering companies, agricultural workers and farmers, many of whom worked on their own with little or no support. To reach these people, the Industrial and Educational committee would set up a meeting of IFFS in a popular location with a speaker, some slides and a video with IFFS leaflets and an invitation to form a small local committee or to join some of the more established committees previously set up. All attending the smaller meetings were invited to the more educational meetings held in the larger centres. As part of its education program, IFFS undertook an extensive programme with Teagasc, the Agricultural Training Authority. Following discussions with John McNamara, Teagasc's health and safety officer, based at Kildalton Agricultural College in south Kilkenny, it was agreed that IFFS personnel would make a series of presentations to students taking the "Green Cert" about eye safety on the farm, in the machine shop and in industries associated with agriculture. In all, 26 individual training centres throughout the country were visited and all students were shown the IFFS campaign video "Lost Horizons".[15] The talks also concentrated on the implications of the Safety, Health and Welfare at Work Act, 1989, for farmers, employees and students, and on the wider ranging social and economic implications of preventable accidents.

IFFS – Hurling Injuries and GAA 1985–2025:

Whereas this injury to Tom Walsh was particularly severe in that he lost an eye, very many of the injuries occurring in hurlers, affected not only the face and eyes, but also other parts of the body. As other parts of the body can be more easily protected, the only protection to the face and head, is with a properly constructed helmet and face gear designed to withstand the collision with a hurley or sliotar ball. On checking with sporting organisations in the US, specially designed head and face protective gear was found to be mandatory in sports such as ice hockey, football, lacrosse, and all sports in which a ball, a racquet or stick could come close to the face and eyes. The Irish Squash Racquets Association also advised the wearing of eye protection when playing squash. The game of cricket has always been associated with the wearing of a high level of protective clothing, including a helmet and faceguard for batsmen at the wicket facing aggressive bowlers.

---

15 Irish Fight for Sight videos: "Lost Horizons". 1988.

Following a publication on hurling injuries by Mr. Philip Cleary, fellow consultant in Waterford Regional Hospital eye department at the time, and Dr. Denise McAuliffe Curtin, ophthalmic surgeon at the Royal Victoria Eye and Ear Hospital in Dublin in 1982, reporting on the growing incidence of facial and eye injuries associated with the sport, a local IFFS committee was set up in Kilkenny.[16]

Eye Injuries Due to Hurling

DENISE McAULIFFE CURTIN
F.R.C.S.I.

PHILIP E. CLEARY
F.R.C.S.

Regional Eye Department
Ardkeen Hospital
Waterford

Irish Medical Journal 1982 "Eye Injuries in Hurling"

Comprising of Larry Hamilton, from Gathabawn, the late Frank Prendergast, Monica Hennessy and others, they began with the job of lobbying local south Kilkenny man, Paddy Buggy, President of the GAA from 1982 to 1985, and prominent officials of the

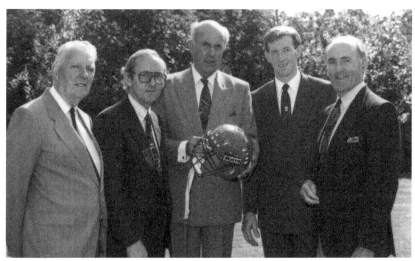

Tom Walsh who lost an eye in the 1967 All Ireland Kilkenny Tipperary Final with Bobby Kerr and John Mitchell (IFFS), Eddie Kerr and Christy Heffernan

---

16 McAuliffe Curtin, D. and Cleary, P, E.: "Eye Injuries Due to Hurling". Irish Medical Journal, Vol. 75, No. 8. 289-290, August 1982

organisation at the time. This resulted in meetings held in Croke Park at GAA headquarters, where they were met with considerable resistance to the wearing of helmets and eye protection.

Meanwhile, they were also in contact with Dr. Michael Loftus, GAA President from 1985 to 1987 through Dr. Ray Niland, a consultant ophthalmic surgeon at Limerick Regional Hospital, who himself had been a GAA football player for Galway. As a GAA member who regularly attended the annual general meetings, Dr. Niland experienced extreme hostility and outspoken criticism from members every time the issue of protection with helmets and eye guards was raised. Finally, after a succession of meetings in Croke Park in GAA HQ, with IFFFS executive, James Kennedy in attendance, the Kilkenny committee received a token agreement that all children, under the age of 12 years, would be advised to wear helmets and face protection. At the time this, represented a disappointment for the committee members, but it did hold out hope that the winds of change might be improving for the future.

In desperation at some of the attitudes of senior members of the GAA, IFFS decided to make a video film, narrated by Mícheál Ó Muircheartaigh, of RTE, on some of the cases that had been encountered over the years, emphasising the need for eye protection for players of the game entitled "Wear the Right Gear".[17] This video was launched by IFFS and the Irish Squash Racquets Association in the spring of 1999 and was supported by major sportsmen of the day including, Nicholas English (Tipperary), and many others. The video helped to provide the basis for all future meetings and was sent out to all the county boards in the country to show to its members.

Finally, in 2010, despite continued failures to debate motions

WEAR THE RIGHT GEAR

**IRISH
FIGHT FOR SIGHT
CAMPAIGN**

*4 Parnell Street
Waterford
Tel: 051 878088
Fax: 051 878606*

---

17 IFFS video "Wear the Right Gear"

put forward at successive AGM's of the GAA on the issue of the use of helmets and face guards for junior and senior players of hurling, the ruling body of the GAA issued the following statement: "The GAA reminds players at all levels in all hurling games and hurling practice sessions, that it is mandatory and the responsibility of each individual player to wear a helmet with a facial guard that meets the standards set out in IS:355 or other replacement standard as determined by the National Safety Authority of Ireland (NSAI). Following the introduction of the rule at underage level, it was proven that mandatory helmet use reduces the number of serious facial and eye injuries by 40%. The rule was introduced across all levels in 2010". Just recently, NSAI announced the updated authenticated specifications for helmet and face guard wear.

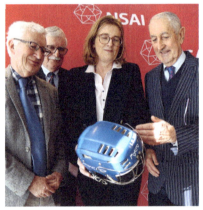

NSAI Helmet Authentication 2025. Lt to Rt: Ray Murray, James Kennedy (IFFS), Angela Larkin (CEO NSAI), Patrick Condon

Nd:YAG Laser Project 1987:

The neodymium YAG laser (Nd:YAG) is a solid state laser developed by Professor Danielle Aron -Rosa, at the Rothschild Institute Clinic in Paris in 1979, which has the capability to disrupt and breakdown dense membranes within the eye without an open surgical procedure. It is extremely useful for opening the residual membrane that sometimes develops after very successful cataract operations and can be done as an outpatient procedure while sitting at a normal examination type slit lamp microscope. In the period before this laser was developed in 1979, the only way in which these membranes could be treated, was mechanically by thrusting a small knife through the front of the eye and physically cutting a hole in the membrane which had to be done in an operating theatre under sterile conditions and was called a capsulotomy operation.

In 1987, I began using the YAG laser for some of our patients in Waterford, by borrowing an instrument from the major company who were selling them at the time. The advantage of this procedure was immediately obvious to the patients, who with just a few eyes drops to expand the pupil of the eye, and the treatment carried out in minutes, had their vision restored fully without the need for hospitalisation and an inpatient surgical procedure. In a report of our initial findings of YAG capsulotomy, approaches were made to the Department of Health for the provision of YAG laser instruments to be made available to the eye unit departments throughout the country with the advantage of obviating the need for the operation of surgical capsulotomy completely.

As the project would undoubtedly involve a significant financial investment by the Dept., the recommendation received quite a negative response. The matter was brought to a head, when RTE approached me to do an item. This resulted in Mr. Kevin McCullough, a farmer from Kilkenny, who had a successful YAG laser treatment in one eye walking out of the unit immediately after treatment without any need for an eye dressing. While this drew some criticism from the Department, and some of my colleague ophthalmologists accused me of advertising and threatened to report me to the Irish Medical Council, it also improved public perception of the major advances and success of modern cataract operations.. The issue was quickly diffused by the IFFS's offer, to all the major eye departments in the country performing surgical capsulotomies, to subsidise half their cost of acquiring these lasers. With the subsequent acquisition by several area health boards and initially the eye departments at University Hospital Galway, the Eye Ear and Throat Hospital Cork, and eye department at Waterford Regional Hospital, it suddenly became standard practice, to phase out the surgical procedure in place of nonsurgical Nd:YAG posterior capsulotomy.

Glaucoma Awareness and Free Testing:

Glaucoma is a disease affecting the eye in which the outward drainage of the fluid from inside the eye is obstructed, resulting in an increase of the internal pressure within the eye which in turn leads to failure in conduction of impulses within the optic nerve which is responsible for transmission of sight to the brain. Because the rise of pressure within the eye occurs very slowly, rarely causing any pain, patients with the problem usually have no symptoms until the sight finally becomes extinguished which is how it got its name of 'Thief in the Night'. The only way in which glaucoma can be diagnosed is by measuring the pressure within the eye using a special measuring device called a tonometer and carried out by either an ophthalmologist, optometrist or glaucoma nurse technician, the normal pressure within the eye averaging 22 mm Hg.

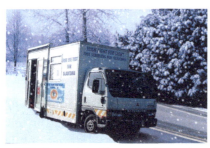

IFFS Campaign Glaucoma Screening Mobile Testing Unit

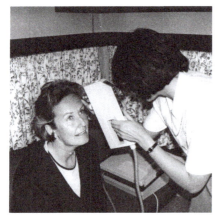

IFFS Campaign Testing for Glaucoma

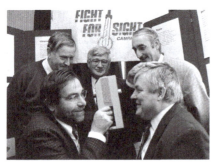

Optometrists Bernard Jennings and others with IFFS Directors Ray Murray and P. Condon

To increase the awareness of glaucoma in the public and to pick up undiagnosed silent cases of glaucoma, IFFS initiated a free testing service for the public with the purchase of a mobile unit fitted out with the necessary equipment for glaucoma testing and staffed with a suitably trained nurse technician to do the testing. The routine involved positioning the unit at a main shopping area in the major towns of the south-east at weekends, where many people could be tested, free of charge, and information leaflets on glaucoma handed out to them. In the case where a person with a raised intraocular pressure was discovered, a note was given to them to have a further test done by their optician who could then refer them to the nearest medical eye centre or hospital eye unit for further management. With time, as the service gather momentum, IFFS, with the help of Mr. Bernard Jennings, Carlow optometrist, started to involve more optometrists in these weekend testing sessions using the IFFS mobile unit. Following a period of free testing for a year, it was found that 12% of patients being tested, had eye pressures over the normal 22 mm Hg and were subsequently referred to medical eye centres, where it was found that 2% suffered from glaucoma. With as much as 2% of the population suffering from undiagnosed glaucoma, the IFFS felt an obligation to continue this service and eventually extended it nationwide.

Sail Around Ireland Fundraising 1991:

Early in 1991, Brian Harris, CEO of IFFS was approached by Mr. Noel Condon, a Westport man living in Dublin, who had gone blind in one eye and was partially sighted in the other from glaucoma. It transpired that the glaucoma had originated from an earlier eye condition at the age of 14 years. As an avid and experienced sailor of small boats, Noel offered to raise money for increased diagnosis and research into glaucoma, by offering to sail single handed around Ireland in his 8-foot boat. On the 23rd of June 1991, with a figure of €30,000 in his head to be raised, Noel Condon set off from Dun Laoghaire harbour, beginning his journey with plans to stop off and visit all major ports around the coast of Ireland on the way. Mr. Brian Harris of IFFS arranged for reception committees to greet him and look after him at all 23 ports around the coast.

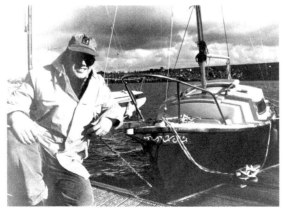

Sail Single Handed Around Ireland – Noel Condon

These reception committees, like those already set up in the south-east by IFFS, and positioned around the coast of Ireland, were also asked to contribute to Noel's effort. For instance, in Westport, where he got an amazing reception, the town arranged The Funny Pram Race, which raised a considerable sum of money. In towns as far west as Castletownbere, following some very heavy weather at sea, he was greeted and hosted as one of their own and given a healthy donation. Having finally completed the 968-nautical mile journey, he returned to Dun Laoghaire Harbour on 28th July with a guaranteed total donation in the region of 100,000 Euros.

Health Board Glaucoma Equipment:

When a patient is diagnosed with glaucoma and put on treatment to lower the pressure in the eye, special tests are needed subsequently to ensure the treatment is effective. This entails the patients having to attend a medical eye clinic for the rest of their lives at intervals for special glaucoma tests. The instrument that is required to do these tests is called a Visual Field Analyser or Perimeter, which checks the full surrounding field of vision in each eye and must be performed by a trained technician. With the increase in glaucoma testing, and a rise in numbers of patients being referred to the Waterford Regional Hospital eye department for glaucoma visual field examinations, it came to the notice of the late Mrs. Maureen Mullins, wife of horse trainer, Paddy Mullins, of Goresbridge, that elderly patients with glaucoma in her area, had to travel from Carlow

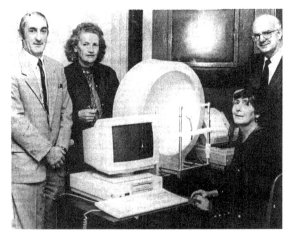

Glaucoma Diagnostic Equipment for SEAHB outpatient-
Maureen Mullins and Rina Cogan (IFFS)

and North Kilkenny to Waterford for these tests and approached the board of IFFS with a fundraising project that would provide these instruments in the Kilkenny and Carlow medical eye clinics for these patients. On consideration by the board, it was decided that this project should be extended to include the clinics in Clonmel, County Tipperary, Wexford and Waterford. Following due consultation with the SEAHB senior health officers, Maureen Mullins and Rina Cogan announced their intention to organise a Special Gala auction in the Carlow / Kilkenny area to provide the necessary instruments for the clinics and set about collecting items of interest for the auction. On the 8th of May 1992, followed by a wine and cheese opening, the IFFS auction began at the Lord Bagenal restaurant in Leighlinbridge with Mr. Fonsie Mealy from Castlecomer, as auctioneer, to conduct the bidding process. Among the items for auction were a nomination to the Bart at Burgage and Ballyhane Studs, a weekend for two in Mount Juliet and several important works of art by contemporary Irish artists. This was followed by a ticket raffle at the end, a total of €26,000 being generated.

National Glaucoma Awareness Week 1993:

With the increased awareness generated by the Sail Around Ireland project and the increased input by optometrists in volunteering to participate in the IFFS free glaucoma testing service in our major towns around Ireland, it was decided to move the programme nationally for a week in July 1993. This was done by writing to all the opticians in the various towns in Ireland requesting their assistance to give free glaucoma testing using the banner of IFFS and sending them glaucoma leaflets to give to those being tested. As well as this, the mobile unit was sent with a driver and its own staff for a half day to each major town extending from Limerick to Galway.

New Frontiers for IFFS 1996 –2004

National Glaucoma Screening Service:

Following the resignation of Mr. Brian Harris from IFFS in 1996, Mr. Bertie Rogers, a retired personnel manager from Waterford Crystal, was appointed chief executive officer and Mrs. Carmel Bolger replaced Ms Marie McSweeney as office secretary. On taking up office, Mr. Rogers in a revision of the logo for the charity, advised the board that the sword of light through the eye and the word Campaign were inappropriate for a caring organisation. It was subsequently agreed for it to be replaced with Irish Fight for Sight. With 12 years in operation and several projects requiring reassessment, Mr. Rogers set about reviewing the free glaucoma screening service. Whereas the service existed on a small scale in the south-east of the country, it was felt that a more nationwide coverage should be targeted. Mr. Rogers and I arranged a meeting in the Department of Health to discuss the feasibility of a free screening service for the country, pointing out that a replacement of the existing mobile unit with funding for a driver and a nurse technician would be required. On emphasising that services provided by optometrists and ophthalmic medical practitioners, would be provided on a voluntary basis, with the advantages of early diagnosis and referral for treatment, as against the threat of blindness from untreated glaucoma, the Department approved a grant of €110,000 to IFFS.

With a new custom-made mobile unit equipped with a state-of-the-art tonometer instrument, the finances available to pay a nurse technician to measure eye pressure, and a driver, the glaucoma screening service started to extend itself throughout the country. This involved the mobile unit with a driver, locating itself at major events, for example, the Royal Dublin Horse Show, race meetings, trade shows and major GAA events, at various locations around the country all year round. It was understood that stand-in optometrists or ophthalmologists for the nurse technician when not available, would provide their services free of charge to IFFS. In spite of this, the running costs of the project which were ongoing, had to be met by continued fundraising much of which came from charity golf competitions organised by Bertie Rogers and Bernard Jennings in Waterford, Tramore and Mount Wolseley in Carlow. By the year 2003, in the previous six months, the unit had travelled to the following towns: Drogheda, Dundalk, Navan, Ennis, Galway, Loughrea, Guinness Dublin, Tallagh, Aer Rianta, Cork, Mallow, Middleton, Killarney, Tralee, Tipperary, Roscrea, Clonmel, Tramore and Waterford. It also attended Galway for the NISO Health and Safety Exhibition and the Diabetes Awareness conference at the RDS in Dublin.

Chapter 16
Eye Bank Ireland 1992–2004

With the growing demand for donor corneal material for transplantation in Ireland, and the increased awareness of organ donation by the Irish Kidney Association based at Beaumont Hospital, it seemed logical that we should establish our own national eye bank for Irish patients. With this in mind, I approached the medical director of the National Blood Transfusion Centre, Mespil Rd., in Dublin, which at the time also housed the National Reference Laboratory and was subsequently referred to the Chief Laboratory Technician, M. Tony Finch, who was most enthusiastic about the project. Following consultation with personal contacts in the Eye Bank of Toronto, Canada about the setting up of an eye bank and a visit to the Corneal Transplant Service Eye Bank (CTS) in Bristol, an application was made to the Department of Health with a project to establish Eye Bank Ireland at the IBTS. This would involve the provision of laboratory space for two technicians who would need to be sent to Bristol to learn the special laboratory techniques used for the preparation of donor corneal material. As designated microscopes and laboratory equipment, incorporating a clean air laminar flow unit, would need to be provided on the return of the technicians who were to set up the bank, an application was made to the Department of Health by the IBTS for funding of the project. While the project was agreed in principle but only feasible within the existing budget of the IBTS, it was considered that part of the cost could be included in the budget allocated to the National Reference Laboratory, the balance to be borne by finances raised privately.

IFFS Eye Bank Funding Campaign Begins:
Since its foundation in 1984, IFFS's major priority in raising awareness of eye injuries and the need for eye protection at work

and at sport, had been largely supported by funds generated from local committees in the south-east of the country and based on the goodwill and care received by relatives of patients attending the unit in Waterford. For instance, Bausch & Lomb employees, at the plant in Waterford, started a donation scheme of one euro per week per employee. Many local committees started to run quizzes in their local social clubs. A well-known board game manufacturer in Waterford designed "Family Quiz" and "My Land" board games for sale at Christmas which were eventually taken over by the "Christmas Cracker" project pioneered by two patients, the late Tom Keene, a retired Garda from Limerick and Nicholas Kirwan from Wicklow, the latter of whom had his sight restored successfully with corneal transplants in both eyes recovered from deceased organ donors through the donation scheme set up at Waterford Regional hospital.

Building on the success of its various projects over the previous seven years since its foundation in 1984, the board of IFFS agreed

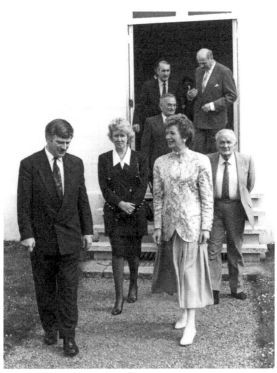

National Eye Bank Opening by President of Ireland, Mary Robinson with Directors of IFFS J. Kennedy, B. Kerr, M. Collins, J, Darrer, J. McGrath, P. Condon

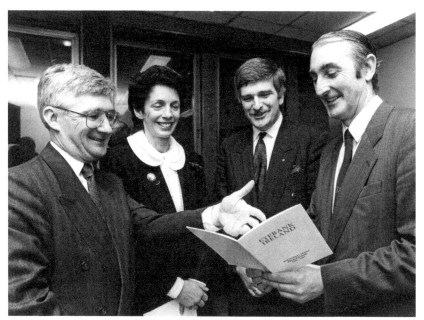
National Eye Bank Programme

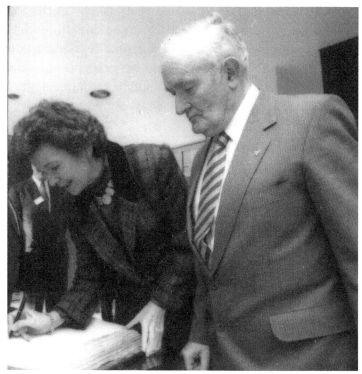
National Eye Bank Opening President of Ireland, Mary Robinson signing the visitors book with Michael Collins

to take on the financing of an Eye Bank project at IBTS in Dublin. Approaches were then made to the IBTS board involving Chief Laboratory Technician, Mr. Tony Finch, which were extremely positive. Having charitable status with a nationwide major health ethos and the attraction of amalgamating with an existing essential medical service (IBTS), an immediate application was made to the National Lottery for funds to support the formation and running costs of an eye bank, Eye Bank Ireland, for a five-year period, after which, consideration would be made by the Department of Health as to its continuation. With due consideration by the National Lottery decision-makers, IFFS was awarded a grant of €252,000.

With initiation of the project by the IBTS, arrangements were made for technician, Ms Sandra Shaw, to work at the Corneal Transplant Service (CTS) in Bristol, UK, where Professor John Armitage had perfected a technique of long term storage of human organ cultured donor corneal material .Plans were immediately put in place to purchase the special equipment required for her on completion of her training. Considering, my close contacts with the Corneal Transplant Service Eye Bank (CTS) in Bristol, and my experience in the setting up of an organ donation scheme at Waterford Regional Hospital, it was agreed by the Department of Health and the IBTS, that I would be available in a medical capacity in the setting up of the bank and be available to the IBTS technical staff for professional advice when required.

See The Light Campaign. Jan. 1992:

With the opening of the Eye bank in late 1992, donated material from Irish hospital became available for use by consultant ophthalmic surgeons in the Republic. With a commitment by IFFS to fund the project for a five-year period at a cost of t €150,000 per year, IFFS decided to launch a nationwide fundraising project in 1993, to highlight the availability of the new national eye bank service at the IBTS in Dublin.

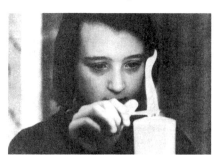

IFFS "See the Light" Campaign with Elizabeth Fardy (Waterford) lighting her candle

Following a reception at the

Áras, by President of Ireland, Mary Robinson, attended by IFFS board representatives, the CEO, Bertie Rogers and company secretary, Mrs. Carmel Bolger, the launching of the "See the Light Week" was planned for Dublin on January 24th, 1993, to run nationally throughout the country for a week ending on January 31st. This involved committees throughout the country being contacted in the months preceding the launch and distributed with See the Light information leaflets about eye donation, and the Eye Bank facility and services. Contacts were made with banks, post offices, unions and public services, requesting them to sell night candles to the public at 1 Euro each and to light them in their homes on the night of 31 January for those people with impairment of sight who might need a transplant in the future and to highlight the need for donations.

The board of IFFS were particularly grateful to successful corneal transplant patients, John O'Reilly from Virginia, Co. Cavan, the late Nicholas Kirwan, from Co. Wicklow, James Martyn Joyce, Renmore, Co. Galway, the parents of teenagers Edel Starkin from Newtownards, Co. Longford and Elizabeth Fardy a 13-year-old from Ferrybank, Waterford, all of whom had received donated corneas through deceased organ donors in the donation scheme at Waterford Regional Hospital and the CTTS service in Bristol. Elizabeth, who had both eyes successfully operated, was honoured by the Lord Mayor of Dunlin, Mr. Sean Kenny TD, with a reception for herself and her family at the Mansion House and later with me was a guest of Pat Kenny on the Late Late Show. On the night of 31st January 1993, the public were asked to light up the candles that they had bought, to celebrate the incoming of spring the following day and the opening of the National Eye Bank service for

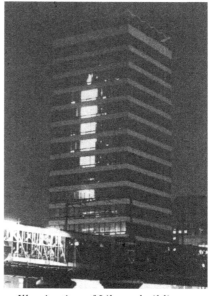

Illumination of Liberty building at Eden Quay Dublin celebrating the "See the Light Campaign"

those rendered blinds from corneal disease who would now have an opportunity to have their sight restored. In a gesture of solidarity, the Liberty building in Dublin was appropriately illuminated with a huge six-story display of a white candle on the front of the building overlooking the river Liffey.

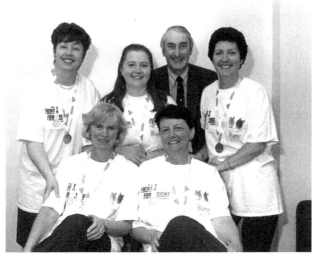

Dept of Ophthalmology" Jennifer Gavin (Right on front row), secretary of the eye department (SEAHB) and IFFS marathon team.

IFFS Eye Bank Ireland Service Commitment 1994–1999:

During the 10-year period after its foundation, Eye Bank Ireland continued to accept ocular tissue donated material from donors countrywide, issuing organ cultured donor material to Irish ophthalmic surgeons. With more surgical indications such as bullous keratopathy, keratoconus, corneal degeneration, corneal trauma or perforation, scarring, ulcers, and chemical burns, requiring healthy donor material, the Eye Bank opened a host of new opportunities for eye surgeons to alleviate blindness from corneal diseases. During the first five years of its existence, Mr. Michael Collins, Managing Director of Clover Meats as an IFFS board member, joined with Mr. Gerry Sheridan, a Dublin accountant and brother to Pat Sheridan of Sheridan Motors, Waterford, to help with the continued fundraising for the bank which was costing €150,000 euros per year. By the end of the fifth year, IFFS had expended €1.5 million on the service, after which the Department of Health took over the management and financial control of the bank.

However, in January 2004, the Eye Bank ceased accepting ocular donations due to concerns surrounding variant Creutzfeldt-Jakob disease (vCJD). As corneas were considered to have a higher theoretical risk of transmission of vCJD than blood, a decision was taken to import all ocular tissue from Rocky Mountain Lions Eye Bank (RMLE) in Denver, Colorado, a vCJD-free zone in the US which still existed up to recently.

Following my retirement as a HSE consultant at Waterford Regional Hospital in 2000, I subsequently offered my resignation as medical director of the Eye Bank. On 12th September 2005, I received a letter from the President of Ireland, Mary McAleese, thanking me for my services as medical director to the National Eye Bank provided over a 20 year period, as well as the services provided at Waterford Regional Hospital and wishing me well in my retirement. (Letter below).

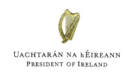

UACHTARÁN NA hÉIREANN
PRESIDENT OF IRELAND

12 September, 2005

Mr. Patrick Condon
Goblin Hill
Grantstown
Co. Waterford

Dear Mr. Condon

It gives me great pleasure to send you my warmest greetings and congratulations on the occasion of your retirement as medical director of the Irish Eye Bank ending almost twenty years of commitment and devotion to restoring sight to many hundreds of people.

Your tireless dedication to the Irish Eye Bank, and to the Waterford Regional Hospital has been a source of inspiration and encouragement to the many people who came into contact with you. You have every right to be very proud of your contribution and achievements.

I am delighted to extend my best wishes to you for a long and happy retirement.

Yours sincerely

Mary McAleese
President of Ireland

Letter from President Mary McAleese on Retirement from Irish Eye Bank Sept 2005

IBTS Tissue Bank and New Eye Bank Ireland – 2008–2025:

The Tissue Bank, based at the Irish Blood Transfusion Service, was licensed by the HPPRA in 2008 to offer a tissue banking service, covering cardiovascular, ocular, skin, and musculoskeletal tissues. In 2021, after a revision of the risk of vCJD transmission through ocular tissue, the possibility of sourcing Irish corneas was reconsidered. As part of the preparation to reopen the Eye Bank, training in-site retrieval has been conducted in the US, with plans to relaunch the retrieval of corneas in Ireland in the fourth quarter of 2025.

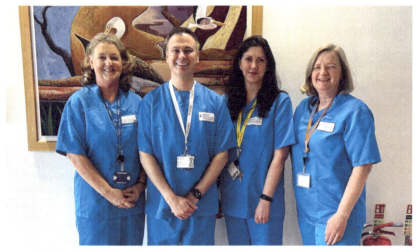

(Left to Right) Sandra Shaw, Chief Medical Scientist, Colin Hynes, Special Medical Scientist, Emma Mc Mahon, Senior Medical Scientist and Beatrix Kelly, Lead Corneal Coordinator.

Chapter 17
IFFS Diabetic Retinopathy Free Screening 2002

Diabetic retinopathy is a condition resulting in leakage of blood into the retina at the back of the eye. It starts with small haemorrhages around the parts of the visual field in the retinal tissue itself, but can become more aggressive, leaking internally and leading to retinal detachment and eventual blindness. Whereas it can occur in all ages, it tends to be more aggressive in younger patients with poorly controlled diabetes. Treatment consists of early intervention, using laser eye treatment and injections into the eye of special medicines. As diabetes is a lifelong disease, it therefore is important that to avoid possible blindness from retinopathy, all diabetics need to be screened by an ophthalmologist from time to time. As this is not possible due to the large numbers of diabetics at all ages, and as many diabetics with early retinopathy can have normal vision without symptoms, a suggested practical solution was the use of a nurse technician with a modern high tech portable retinal camera to obtain photographs of each patient.

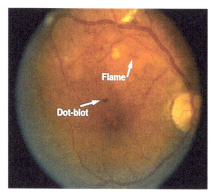

Diabetic retinopathy showing early haemorrhaging at the back of the eye

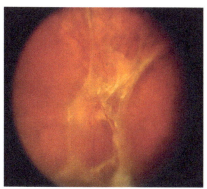

Advanced diabetic retinopathy following major eye haemorrhage

Subsequent examination of the obtained photos could then be interpreted by an offsite ophthalmologist not unlike the system employed by radiologists. Patients found to have retinopathy would then be referred straight to the special retinal clinic for possible treatment. For maximum convenience and to encourage attendance, it seemed that the most convenient place for this to take place was in the patients' general practitioner practice. In consultation with some of the larger general practices in the south-east as to the provision of an in-house screening service for their patients, there was unanimous acceptance of the idea.

Subsequently, I approached IFFS with a project to purchase a portable digital Topcon non-mydriatic digital retinal camera and to set up a pilot scheme offering a free screening service to the general practices in the south-east area with large numbers of diabetics. The service would be operated by an eye trained nurse technician and results from a photographic session sent electronically to a computer in my office for screening. The general practitioners would then be informed of the identity of the patients with retinopathy which allowed them to refer them onwards for treatment. At first, it was felt that the IFFS office should be responsible for organisation of the service with the general practitioners directly. With full approval from the board of IFFS, the pilot project was arranged initially with a major practice in the New Ross district, which proved to be extremely successful in that most if not all the patients lived in the surrounding area, obviating the need to travel to Waterford. Within two years, we covered the major general practices in the south-east such as the Walsh practice in new Ross, the Keogh practice in Waterford, the Cuddihy practice in Kilkenny and many others in the Carlow, Wexford and South Tipperary areas.

After a period of two years of success, the Diabetic Retinopathy Free Service was launched by President of Ireland, Mary McAleese in Waterford on 11th June, June 2004. This was combined with presentations by the President to the volunteer committee members of IFFS. Thirteen years later, the HSE announced the introduction of a National Diabetic Retinopathy Screening Service in 2013 with the setting up of special screening centres around the country at which trained technicians with their equipment screen patients for the general practitioners, the results being electronically monitored.

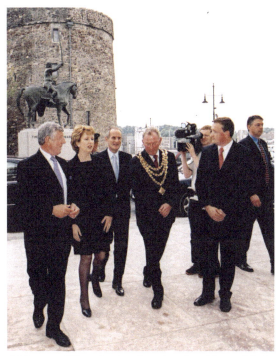

IFFS and Mayor of Waterford welcoming President of Ireland Mary McAleese for the launch of the IFFS Diabetic Retinopathy Free Screening Service

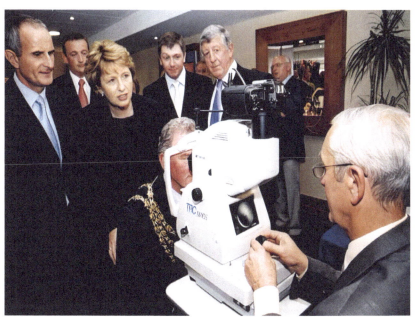

Mayor of Waterford being tested using the advanced Non Mydriatic Retinal camera

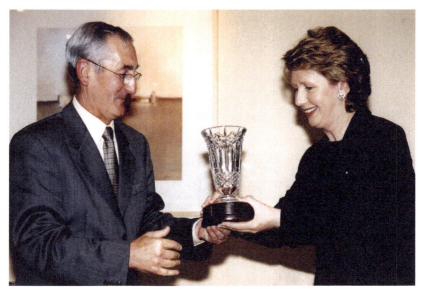

Mr. Patrick Condon receiving a presentation from President of Ireland, Mary McAleese

IFFS National Conference on Eye Protection – "A Lot to Lose", 2003:

A major conference took place on March 6th, 2003, at the Green Isle Hotel in Dublin, which was the first of its type in Ireland focusing on the prevention of sight loss. The theme for the conference was designed to address screening for eye diseases, the way in which eye injuries occur and more importantly, ways in which they can be prevented in the workplace, in sport and in the home. The conference was opened by Mr. Michael Ahern TD, Minister for Trade and Commerce and was supported by the Health and Safety Authority and NISO. In her opening address,

Fight For Sight
4 Parnell Street,
Waterford
Tel: 051 878088

A Lot To Lose II
Running Time 20min

Crystal Productions
Tel: 051 895 490

IFFS Video Label - A Lot to Lose II

the chairperson Mary Darling stated "Our eyes are our window on the world and without sight we would live in a dark place. They are precious and irreplaceable". At the opening of the event, a new video and CD-rom "*A Lot to Lose 11*" was launched.[18] As well as covering a huge range of enacted scenes and situations of accidents and the ways in which they occur, it was interspersed with interviews by the health and safety organisations. This video had already been used by a wide number of companies throughout the country promoting aspects of health and safety. The conference was well attended by safety officers from the major companies, small engineering companies and representatives from the safety organisations. It also featured a huge exhibition of safety equipment for all aspects of industry, agriculture and included in particular the full range of protective head and facial gear available for participation in the sport of hurling.

Funding for the conference was raised by means of a dinner and auction at the Four Seasons Hotel in Dublin in September organised by the Confederation of Optical Suppliers Ireland (COSI). Organisers of the event included John Macklin, President of COSI, Deirdre O'Sullivan and Suzanne Berne, together with Bernard Jennings, Chairman of the IFFS board and Rachel Tracey, Director of IFFS, including Catherine Belton, who facilitated the event at the hotel. One of the highlights of the auction, was a painting by the late Tony O'Malley, which was kindly presented by his wife Jane. The bidding reached fever pitch with the mallet coming down on €36,000. Other highlights were the performances of Barry Murphy and Pauline McGlynn.

IFFS 2004–2017:

Since its formation in 1984, IFFS had witnessed a remarkable decline in the incidence of severe eye injuries during its 20-year history. With the help of updated state legislation in all aspects of health and safety, and increased emphasis on the value of sight and the provision of eye protection in motorised transportation, industry and agriculture, progress had been remarkable. Whereas many of the changes were welcomed by the major organisations for reasons of liability, DIY workers and those working in isolated situations, were quite reluctant at first to become involved,

---

18 Irish Fight for Sight video "A Lot To Lose 11", 2003.

but finally made the changes necessary to protect employees in their place at work. The reticence to the wearing of head and eye protection for 30 years by the GAA, before finally making them mandatory in 2010, was a classic example of long-term pressure strategy that in the end prevailed.

The introduction by IFFS of the free screening schemes, not only brought the hidden dangers of sight loss from undiagnosed glaucoma and diabetic retinopathy to the attention of the public but also promoted the early diagnosis of these conditions with referral for treatment before significant sight loss. By 2013, testing for glaucoma had become part of a standard eye test for glasses carried out by optometrists throughout the country with the advantage of early diagnosis and referral for treatment. Meanwhile, the IFFS diabetic retinopathy screening initiated in the south-east, was finally replaced by a state funded National Diabetic Retinopathy Screening service embracing the whole country.

With the opening of the eye surgical unit in Waterford in 1976, and the setting up of the corneal service, the concept of the deceased organ donor scheme for corneal transplantation was established. Working with the Irish Kidney Association in the retrieval of donated material resulting from fatal accidents and their donor card promotional material, the concept of eye donation became synonymous with the national organ donation programme. As the numbers of successful corneal transplant patients increased in the 1980s, with the demand for more donations, the need for the Eye Bank became much more essential where donations could be stored safely for longer periods and if not used in Ireland for some reason, could be donated to the UK and central Europe Eye Banks through international cooperative arrangements. Whereas the launch of the National Eye Bank at IBTS in January 1993 and the subsequent funding for five years was a daunting undertaking by the directors of IFFS, its continued success in the restoration of sight for a further 10 years will not be forgotten.

IFFS International Contribution:
Asante Eye Clinic Kenya:

With his continuous and generous contribution over the years in the setting up of the free glaucoma screening service and in engaging the support of optometrists for the activities of IFFS, Mr.

Bernard Jennings, Carlow optometrist, as chairman of the board in 2003, introduced the Asante project in the Eastern Province of Kenya. The project involved a screening for eye disease for the Wakamba population in a remote missionary area in Kenya run by Irish Mercy nuns, several of whom were from the Carlow area. Whereas a basic health facility was being currently undertaken by the nuns, there did not appear to be any form of eye service available in the area. The project involved qualified eye personnel from Ireland travelling to Nairobi, followed by an 8-hour cross country jeep drive with the purpose of carrying out eye examination clinics in Asante and the villages in the surrounding area. Following their first visit, Mr. Jennings and his fellow colleague optometrists who journeyed there, soon discovered the total lack of adequate equipment for eye examination and testing. With donations from the optometric profession and funding from IFFS, ophthalmoscopes and optical examination microscopes were provided during several visits. The screening process involved eye testing for glasses. Patients with eye diseases such as cataracts, glaucoma, and damaged eyes from infection and accidents, were referred to the eye hospital in Nairobi for treatment by consultant eye surgeons. As each visit by Bernard and colleague were usually limited to a week including travelling, they still managed to see 6,000 people, 800 of which were referred on for treatments over a 10-year period.

Ile a Vache Eye Clinic Haiti:

Founded in 2015, Irish ophthalmologist Dr. Kevin Tempany set up a sustainable eye clinic for indigenous people with local ophthalmologists and optometrists providing a community based eyecare service on the south coast of Haiti Island.

IFFS Dissolution 31st July, 2017 – Announcement:

1. "Thirty-three years on from its foundation, the Board of Fight for Sight decided to implement a gradual winding down of the charity's activity. The decision was tinged with sadness, but consolation was taken from the knowledge that the objectives set out in 1984 had been achieved and that the charity had made very significant

contributions in the fields of preservation and protection of eyesight. The winding down process was to conform with standard charitable legislation. This includes the distribution of all remaining funds to other sight charities and to international eyecare clinics which Fight for Sight already supported. These include:

2. World Sight Foundation: Established in 2012, the foundation's mission is to deliver sustainable solutions for the alleviation of blindness, and for preserving sight anywhere in the world. While the Foundation is not involved with the direct provision of services, it is instead focused on enhancing the skills of locally-based eyecare professionals through education.
3. Asante Project – Kenya
4. Ile A Vache – Haiti.

Chapter 18
"Freedom from Glasses"

Refractive Surgery – Lasik and PRK:

Refractive surgery is surgery on the eye with the purpose of altering its optical power and the shape of the pathways of light entering and exiting from the eye. The term is also used in the correction of short and long sightedness, thereby obviating the need for glasses or contact lenses. The cornea, or front window of the eye, not only transmits light rays and images passing through to the retina or "film" at the back of the eye but also acts as a focusing lens to sharpen these images, so that the retina can visualise these images clearly. Whereas the shape of the cornea and its focusing power in the normal cornea are fixed, the length of the eyeball itself can vary from person to person as in myopia or short-sightedness and hyperopia or long sightedness. In persons with these shortcomings, the use of glasses and contact lenses are generally used to normalise sight. In those who do not wish to wear glasses, refractive surgery involves flattening or steepening of the cornea to change the focusing effect on the retina.

Keratomileusis:

In 1948, José Ignacio Barraquer in Bogotá, South America produced his thesis on The Law of Corneal Thicknesses: "That cornea flattens when tissue is removed from the centre of the cornea and steepness when tissue is removed from the periphery". To prove his point, he invented a surgical instrument called the microkeratome which could be applied surgically to the surface of the eye, to remove a thin

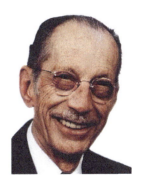

Dr. José Ignacio Barraquer

slice of surface cornea which was machined in a specially adapted sterile lathe to thin it and reapply it to the eye of the patient. This operation for myopia or short-sightedness was called keratomileusis and was subsequently taken up by Krumeich in Germany and Swinger in the US, who modified the instrument and the technique. However with the technical difficulties using the microkeratome in performing the refractive cut and removing the excised piece of cornea, this procedure was considered too difficult and abandoned.

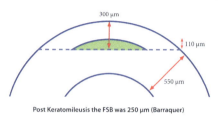

The operation of Keratomileusis (excised piece of corneal tissue in green)

Radial Keratotomy:

In 1974, Prof Svyatoslav Fyodorov, at the National Institute of Research in Moscow, USSR, introduced the operation of Radial Keratotomy for the correction of myopia, which involved deep radially placed corneal incisions to flatten the cornea which he promoted worldwide as the Russian operation. However with the publication of the Prospective Evaluation of Radial Keratoty (PERK) 10 year report, which highlighted the long term complications, RK was discontinued.

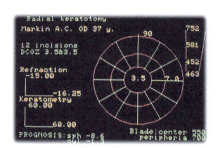

The operation of Radial Keratotomy

Automated Lamellar Keratoplasty:

Meanwhile, in Bogotá, Colombia, South America, Barraquer's microkeratome had been totally redesigned by Dr. Luis Antonio Ruiz. Because of its major surgical and technical advantages over the original completely manual Barraquer microkeratome, it was called the Automated Corneal Shaper (ACS). The surgical term of " keratomileus" for the procedure was also changed to Automated Lamellar Keratoplasty (ALK). This modified instrument manufactured in Florida by Steinway Medical, was marketed by Chiron who were organising courses throughout the United

States by Dr. Charles Casebeer. Having attended a number of his courses on ALK, which included hands on wet laboratory practice with the ACS, the value of the instrument to perform partial thickness or lamellar corneal transplantation, seemed to have great advantages. In order to familiarise myself more with the ALK procedure, I arranged to travel to Bogotá and spend two days visiting Dr. Ruiz, to observe him operate and review his patients post operatively

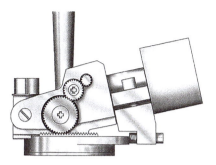

The Automated Lamellar Keratotomy System

With the increased growth of interest in the correction of myopia in Europe and the acquisition of an ACS instrument for the corneal transplant work we were doing in Waterford, we started to incorporate lamellar or partial thickness corneal transplantation into our services. As part of training for the doctors from the different countries working as senior house officers and at registrar level with us at the time, a room in the eye department was set aside as a wet laboratory area for them to practice their surgical skills on recovered abattoir pigs eyes.

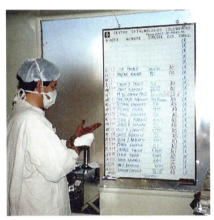

Dr. Luis Antonio Ruiz observing his operating theatre list

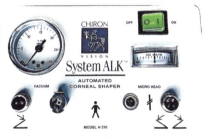

The Automated Corneal Shaper Microtome Instrument (ACS)

Photo refractive Keratectomy:

Following research by Dr. Stephen Trokel in the US and Prof John Marshall at the Institute of Ophthalmology in London in the early '80s, on the suitability of different wavelengths of excimer laser light to remove tissue from the surface of the cornea, the excimer laser instrument was approved for use to treat myopia, the term, "photo refractive keratectomy" (PRK) being coined. PRK was first introduced into Ireland by Dr. Frank Lavery, the owner of the Wellington eye clinic in Dublin in the early '80s, followed by Prof Michael O'Keeffe at the Mater Hospital eye clinic and Temple Street Children's Hospital in Dublin, where it was used in the treatment of amblyopia in children with unilateral short or long sightedness. With the establishment of the Summit European customer care and maintenance facility in Cork at about the same time, both centres benefited greatly with newly developed laser algorithms and upgrades to their equipment.

Lasik and the Mater Hospital Laser Clinic Development: 1989

On October 25th 1989, Dr. Lucio Buratto, in Milan, Italy repeated the original surgery by Barraquer removing a corneal flap with an original Barraquer microkeratome on a patient, followed by a PRK excimer laser treatment on the stromal surface of the excised tissue and replacing it on the patients eye. The following year, Dr. Ioannis Pallikaris from Crete, Greece, was the first to apply PRK excimer laser treatment to the exposed patient's stroma under a prepared hinged flap, using an original Barraquer microkeratome. It was with the support of the Summit laser company and Chiron, manufacturers of the ACS microkeratome, that motivated Professor O'Keeffe and myself, to carry out our first laser in-situ keratomileusis

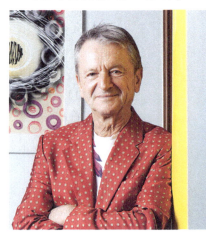

Professor Dr. Lucio Buratto, Ambrosia Clinic, Milan

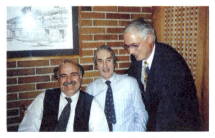

Professor Ioannis Pallikaris, Jorg Krumeich and P. Condon

procedure on 17th March, 1990, at the Mater Hospital in Dublin, in which we used the ACS with an ALK procedure to produce a hinged corneal flap followed by a PRK treatment on the exposed stromal bed, replacing the flap without suturing. To my knowledge, this was one if the first recorded ALK-PRK procedure carried out in Ireland and the UK at the time. Almost immediately, the term laser in situ keratomileusis was universally changed to the shortened version of Lasik. In recognition of this work, in the same year, I was awarded the Montgomery Medal Lecture by the Irish College of Ophthalmology for my presentation entitled "Refractive Surgery – A Replacement for Spectacles" which took place in Trinity College, Dublin in 1990.

Following significant success with this combination of PRK laser treatment and the ACS microkeratome, I approached the programme manager for hospitals (SEAHB) with a project to refer highly myopic patients with a disability for me to treat at the clinic in Dublin on an outpatient sessional basis. An arrangement was made by the SEAHB and the Mater Hospital for me to attend on a monthly basis to carry out a Lasik operating list on patients from the south-east, beginning at 8 am, for which I

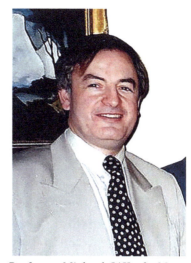

Professor Michael O'Keefe, Mater Hospital Laser Clinic, Dublin

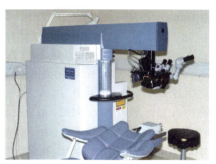

Summit Excimer Laser

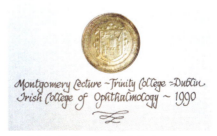

Irish College of Ophthalmology Montgomery Medal 1990

would bring the pre-sterilised ACS microkeratome and instruments with me.

We then continued with operations on a series of highly myopic patients using ultrasound pachymetry to measure the thickness of the cornea as we progressed. While in most cases, it was not possible to correct the degree of short-sightedness fully because of the strict limitations on the amounts of tissue that could be removed safely, the reduction in the extreme degrees of short-sightedness, was nevertheless of considerable advantage to these patients postoperatively in improving their sight and reducing their disability. At the European Intraocular Implant Council (EIIC) meeting in Gothenburg in 1996, I presented our 6 year results which were subsequently reported in the Ophthalmology in 1997.[19]

With the rapid demand for refractive surgery by the public worldwide, the instrument and laser technology companies began to produce a range of new products, some of which were available on short-term loans from the companies. This provided an opportunity for the laser clinic to upgrade the existing equipment. As a result, the long-standing ACS microkeratome was replaced by a fully automated Summit Krumeich Barraquer Microkeratome (SKBM) system. The Summit laser was initially replaced by the Aesculap Meditec Mel 60 eximer laser, a similar laser system to the one used at the time by Professor Ioannis Pallikaris at the University of Crete, Greece, where Michael and I attended

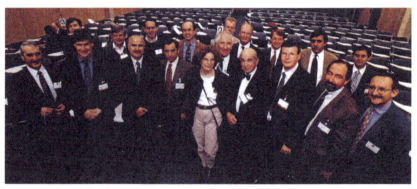

ESCRS Lasik Working group Symposium Gothenburg 1996

---

19 Condon P.I., Mulhern M., Fulcher, T., Foley-Nolan A, O'Keefe, M: "Laser Intrastromal Keratomileusis for High Myopia and Myopic Astigmatism" Ophthalmology; 81:199-206,1997.

EUROPEAN SOCIETY OF
CATARACT AND REFRACTIVE SURGEONS
(Formerly EIIC)

10 Hagan Court, Lad Lane,
Dublin 2, Ireland
Tel: 353-1-6618904 Fax: 353-1-6785047

Correspondence to:-

EUROPEAN LAMELLAR KERATOPLASTY USERS GROUP

DATE: Tuesday, 20th September 1994.
TIME: 7.00am - 9.00am
LOCATION: Lecture Theatre 'E', FIL Congress Centre.

10 minute presentation, 5 minute dicussion
Coffee and orange juice will be served

07.00	Comparision of P.R.K. and KM in high myopia - K. Williams (United Kingdom).
07.15	Automated Lamellar Keratoplasty step by step: The role of Chiron/Steinway corneal shaper. - M. Zirm (Austria) - Video.
07.30	Initial Results of automated lameller keratoplasty with LASIK using the Technolas excimer laser. - J. Guell (Spain).
07.45	Excimer Laser KM in the treatment of myopia. - T. Salah (Saudi Arabia).
08.00	Complications of LASIK. - I. Pallikaris (Greece).
08.15	Critical evaluation of ALK in comparsion to other techniques of correction for high myopia. - G. O. Waring (USA).
08.30	Complications of ALK. - D. Lebuisson (France).
08.45	Initial experiences with ALK with/without excimer laser: What the experts did not tell us..... - P. I. Condon/M. O'Keefe (Ireland).

09.00 - 09.30 Formation of European Users Group

President: PHILIPPE SOURDILLE France, *Secretary:* ULF STENEVI Sweden, *Treasurer:* PATRICK CONDON Ireland
Board members: PETER BARRY Ireland, MICHAEL BLUMENTHAL Israel, LUCIO BURATTO Italy, LEIF CORYDON Denmark, GUNTHER GRABNER Austria
DANIEL LEBUISSON France, THOMAS NEUHANN Germany, JOHN PEARCE United Kingdom, BO PHILIPSON Sweden, EMANUEL ROSEN United Kingdom

ESCRS Gothenburg Lasik Symposium Program

the Meditec training course and reviewed some of his patients. Because of increasing developments in laser technology, a Chiron Technolase 116-117 laser system was then installed which was subsequently upgraded, to the Bausch and Lomb Technolase 217. While both Professor O'Keeffe and myself continued to carry out standard refractive Lasik surgery on our patients, Michael became actively involved in the paediatric side of things, publishing extensively on Lasik in children and paediatric refractive surgery

European Society of Cataract and Refractive Surgery – Evolution

European Intraocular Implant Council (EIIC) 1982–1993:

The European Intraocular Implant Council was set up in 1982 by Dr. Cornelius Binkhorst with a board of officers all of whom were European lens implant surgeons. When news got out, that we in Ireland had been routinely carrying out modern cataract and lens implant surgery since 1976, I was contacted by Cornelius Binkhorst and invited to become the Irish member representative on his newly founded European Intraocular Implant Council (EIIC) which offered me the opportunity to make a presentation at their upcoming first European meeting at The Hague in September 1982. At the meeting, I presented a joint paper with my registrar, Dr. H. Zalzalla, entitled *"Intraocular Pressure Lowering Techniques for Cataract Surgery"*.

The second meeting a year later in 1983 was organised by Professor Karl Jacobi in Giessen, with the help of the German national implant society, followed a year later in 1984 by a meeting in Harrogate, UK organised by David Bowan and Piers Percival of UKIOIS. In 1985, Dr. Leo Anar in conjunction with the French intraocular lens implant society, organised an excellent meeting in Cannes, southern France, which was followed by a gap of two years, during which membership was extended to Emanuel Rosen from the UK and who started to participate in the early committees with which I had already become involved. As it was extremely difficult to communicate with other members due to the various language differences, I was delighted to have a UK colleague join the membership for support. In 1986, I was appointed to the board of the EIIC and attended the meeting in Jerusalem, Israel, in 1987 organised by Professor Michael Blumenthal and the Israeli Implant Society. Having attended the previous three meetings and with my position on the board, I developed a strong feeling of empathy for the organisation and made many friends while all the time improving my diplomatic skills. In 1987, Emanuel Rosen took over as president of the EIIC from Binkhorst with a view to possibly make major changes within the Council which he felt he could not accomplish by himself. As a result, he surrounded himself with a core group of allies, Ulf Stenevi from Sweden, Michael Blumenthal from Israel and myself from Ireland. One aspect that had to be tackled, was in relation to the independent organisation of the annual conference by the individual national societies in the country in which they were held and the degree of their accountability to the EIIC. During the next two years, together with other enthusiasts, and with a goal to include refractive surgeons in the council, the theoretical name of the European Society of Cataract and Refractive Surgeons was born. In 1988, Ulf Stenevi and Bo Philipson with the national Swedish implant society, organised the EIIC meeting in Copenhagen followed a year later in 1989 in Zurich, Switzerland, organised by Dr. Schimmelpfening and the Swiss implant society. With possible amalgamation of the national societies under a single European organisation, Rosen also proposed that in such a situation, a secretariat would need to be considered. During this period, while new ideas were being floated around, I volunteered to organise the next conference in Dublin in 1990.

"Major Conference for Dublin" –
1990 EIIC Annual Conference:

Having just two years to organise a major conference seemed to me at the time a crazy decision in view of the fact that as President of the Irish Ophthalmological Society (IOS), I was heavily involved in negotiating the amalgamation of the Irish Society with the Irish Faculty of Ophthalmologists, to form the new Irish College of Ophthalmologists (ICO). Nevertheless, the boost to Irish ophthalmology in bringing a major European society meeting to Dublin seemed a worthwhile challenge at the time. Being the only Irish EIIC member in Ireland and without a national implant society, it fell to me to organise the business and scientific aspects of the conference. Having worked with Peter Barry as secretary of the IOS in the formation of the new College, and with his known reputation of "getting things done", I asked him if he would be interested in getting involved. Little did we realise that his decision to become involved at this stage would win him, the Presidency of the ESCRS in 2012.

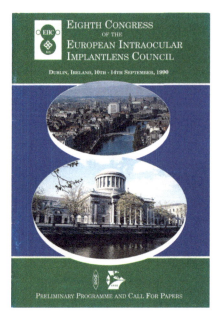

EIIC 8th Annual Congress, Dublin, 1990

EIIC Council Membership, 1990

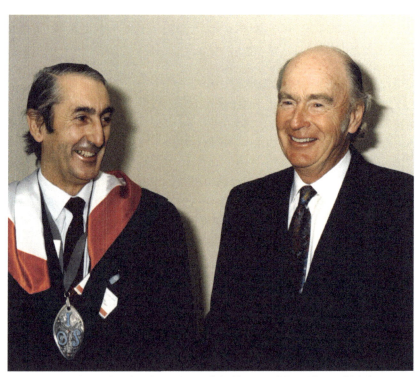

President of Ireland, Dr. Patrick Hillary and President of Irish Ophthalmological Society, Dr. Patrick Condon at the Opening of EIIC Conference, Dublin, 1990

Together with Peter, who was a consultant vitreoretinal surgeon at St. Vincent's Hospital and the Royal Victoria Eye and Ear Hospital in Dublin, we decided to advertise for a conference organiser and were most lucky to come in contact with Mrs. Mary Dardis who had worked with the Department of Public Health and had just set up an event management conference organising company in Dublin called Agenda Communications and Conference Services. At an interview with Agenda in the boardroom of the Royal Victoria Eye and Ear Hospital in Dublin, Peter Barry and myself signed a contract with them to organise the conference in Trinity College, College Green, Dublin to be held on the 10th September, 1990. With my eight year experience of EIIC contacts in Europe and the US through the Irish American Ophthalmological Society, our first job was to write a letter to the officers of all the European national implant societies and the American Society of Cataract and Refractive Surgeons (ASCRS) to enter it into their calendar of future meetings while Agenda booked Trinity College as the venue for the conference.

During the subsequent year, while attending many of the European and American meetings, Peter Barry and myself heavily promoted the conference at the various sub committee meetings and social events. While doing our day job and on call for our hospitals, dealing with the politics and formation of the new Irish College and meetings with Agenda regarding organisational details of the conference, many late evenings were spent in Peter and Carmel Barry's house with late-night commutes from Dublin to Waterford for me or sometimes overnighting in Dublin with an early morning meeting there the next day. When it came to reviewing the abstracts and preparation of the scientific programme, there was no large committee to help, which in many ways, was probably an advantage in that discussion was minimal and decisions efficiently made. One of the aspects that had not been included in any previous EIIC conference was a morning of live surgery at St Vincent's Hospital which Peter Barry organised with his colleagues there.

The opening ceremony of the conference at the National Concert Hall was attended by the President of Ireland, Dr. Patrick Hillary, the Minister for Health, Dr. Rory O'Hanlon, Harold Ridley, Congress President, his wife Elizabeth and myself as

President of the Irish Ophthalmological Society. Harold Ridley presented the Ridley Medal to John Marshall for his lecture on "Recent Advances in Excimer Laser Surgery" and Mrs. de Jonge presented the Kiewiet de Jonge award to Jan Worst, of the Netherlands. This was then followed at Trinity College by a varied scientific programme covering all aspects of intraocular lens implant surgery and was extremely well supported by the instrument and pharmaceutical companies. One of the key events enjoyed by all, was the conference dinner held in the magnificent surroundings of Dublin Castle. Apart from the usual social events occurring at these meetings, in acknowledgement to Emanuel Rosen as president of the EIIC, the Royal College of Surgeons in Ireland awarded him an honorary FRCS (Ire.) at a function in the college on Stephen's Green. As well as attending the conference, many delegates who had never visited Ireland previously, also enjoyed the various hospitality tours organised by Agenda to different parts of the country.

Dublin – European Headquarters "Agenda Communications" 1993–2023:

With eight increasingly successful annual congresses, each independently organised by individual national societies for the EIIC, the very successful organisation of the Dublin conference with the use of an independent professional event management company, appealed to Emanuel Rosen.

At a subsequent meeting of officers of the Council, he recommended, that based on the excellent result of the Dublin meeting, and the imminent formation of the European Union to oversee the economic and political integration by all members of the European Community in 1993, that a central English-speaking European office for the society with organisational

Mary Dardis, Agenda Communications, Dublin, Ireland

capabilities, be set up within the European Union for the EIIC. Whereas several of the existing national implant societies applied for the opportunity to develop the centralised office for the Council in their own countries, it was decided that the central office and organisational system capabilities offered by Agenda Communications in Dublin, would be the most satisfactory arrangement both financially and politically. As a result, it was agreed to outsource to an event management company with office facilities to provide conference and office services for a five-year time span starting in 1991 and located in Dublin. Several companies tendered for the position, but Agenda with their years of office experience and organisational ability, were chosen and offered a five-year contract by the EIIC.

Chapter 19
Formation of European Society of Cataract and Refractive Surgeons – Dublin 1991–1993

The transformation of the European Council to a European Society, incorporating refractive surgery in its name, was spearheaded by Emanuel Rosen as president. With legal contacts in London, he set up a company structure with limited liability and charity registered with the Charities Commission in the United Kingdom.

> "The society is governed by bylaws agreed by the members. These bylaws are updated from time to time to serve the needs of the society. The general management of the society is vested in an elected Board, members of which includes the president, secretary, treasurer, president elect, directors of the society, editor of the Journal of Cataract and Refractive Surgery and 10 ordinary members. Elections to the Board are held every two years. Board members serve a term of four years and may be elected for one additional term. The Board of the ESCRS elects a president for a term of two years. No more than one ordinary member of the board may be from the same country. From time to time the board co-opts additional members nominated by their national societies to represent important membership groups that are otherwise not represented.

> An executive committee consisting of the president, president-elect, secretary, and treasurer ensure that the decisions of the board are implemented.

> The Board is assisted by six standing committees: Finance, General purposes, Programme, Research, Publications and

Education. The Board may form additional ad hoc committees that it considers necessary.

Full membership of the society is confined to European ophthalmologists. Group membership is open to European national society members, and such members are entitled to full membership rights, including voting rights."[20]

New Irish ESCRS Treasurer and Congress Committee Chairperson Appointments 1991–1999:

With the success and experience of Dublin behind us, and the funds generated by the congress going to the EIIC instead of a national implant society, it was decided by the EIIC Council in the interest of the future consolidation of its resources, that the finance and congress committees be amalgamated under a single chairmanship. As an EIIC Council and Board member with a track record of attending all previous meetings since its foundation in 1982, and involved in the Dublin conference organisation, I was asked by the EIIC Council to take responsibility for the financial aspect of the ESCRS as treasurer and to chair the Congress committee which could provide the bulk of funds to the society from the annual conference, which I accepted. As I had been extremely happy with the firm of accountants that we appointed for the Dublin conference, it was a great comfort to me in this new position for them to be reappointed as the accountants for the ESCRS. Two subsequent conferences were held, one in Valencia, Spain (1991), and the other in Paris, France (1992) under the auspices of the EIIC with Emanuel as the first president of the ESCRS. Emanuel's successor, Philip Sourdille as president and together with Dan Lebuisson who organised the Paris conference, had the unenviable task of introducing the decision by the Board to implement English as the official language of the society, which for the French and Italian delegates attending the conference, necessitated facilities for simultaneous translation, which added an extra financial burden to the meeting. This was followed by Innsbruck, Austria (1993), Lisbon, Portugal (1994), Amsterdam, the Netherlands (1995), Gothenburg, Sweden (1996), Prague, the

---

20 "About the ESCRS" Appendix 1, European Soc. of Cataract and Refractive Surgeons – A History by Emanuel Rosen and Peter Barry Page 117, 2013.

Czech Republic (1997), Nice, French Rivera (1998) and Vienna (1999), under successive presidents, Michael Blumenthal (Israel), and Thomas Neuhann (Germany) all of which were organised directly by the Congress committee.

Congress Trade Exhibition Companies:

Because ophthalmology involves large elements of instrumental and pharmaceutical diagnostic and therapeutic products, attendance at congresses is the only way in which companies can showcase their products conveniently to a large group of ophthalmologists in a relatively short period of time. As a result, there was always a continuous interest in the companies to become actively involved and for the ESCRS congress committee, this became an extremely important issue. Whereas the provision of exhibition space and facilities for these companies to exhibit their products was extremely expensive, funding generated by these congresses when combined with the delegates registration fees could accumulate considerably. In the case of the ESCRS Congress committee, these monies were then allocated to the Finance committee to be used for the scientific, research and educational aspects of cataract and refractive surgery. Another aspect that facilitated the rapid development of the society in the early days, was the considerable delay in approval by the FDA in the United States of American made products for sale in the US market, which provided an impetus for American companies to market their products in Europe where EMA approval was less formidable.

All the organisations involved in staging these meetings might give rise to the impression that an overwhelming amount of personal effort was required. However, having the central office in Dublin with the staff and expertise of Agenda to carry the administrative burden, an active scientific program committee set up by the ESCRS Board, and competent accountants to deal with the finances, routine conference business was largely dealt with by telephone conferencing and email. However, for major planning ahead and accountancy reasons, full executive meetings with the chairpersons of the committees were usually held at the end of each year at head-quarters in Dublin and in the middle of the following year prior to the annual congress. As well as keeping me in close contact with the intimate workings of all aspects of the society, this arrangement allowed me to continue my full schedule of work for the SEAHB at Waterford Regional Hospital.

Journal of Cataract and Refractive Surgery and Eurotimes:

With his experience as editor of the European Journal of Implant and Refractive Surgery for the EIIC, and its publication in Paris prior to the formation of the ESCRS, Emanuel Rosen was quick to start the Publication committee. Supported by Philip Sourdille who had a research interest to inject a more scientific impetus into the society, a proposition was put forward for an amalgamation of the American Journal of Cataract and Refractive Surgery (JCRS) with the European Journal. As each ESCRS Congressed meeting progressed and considerable profits accumulated, a proposition was put to the Finance committee to fund the project. Following long, lengthy discussions with Dr. Stephen Obstbaum, editor of the JCRS and David Karcher, CEO of the ASCRS, with particular reference as to how much investment would be required by both societies, an agreement was finally reached resulting in the current Journal. Tributes were paid to the work of both Douglas Koch (US) and Thomas Kohnen (Germany) for their combined effort in maintaining the flow of reviewed manuscripts while negotiations were in progress.

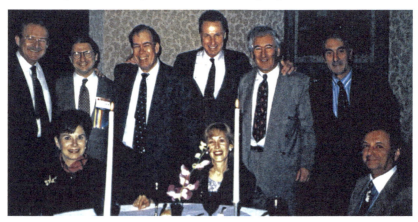

Merger of ESCRS and ASCRS Journals to form the Journal of Cataract and Refractive Surgery (JCRS) Front row Lt to Rt: Merill Obsbaum, Anne Kelman, Charlie Kelman. Back Row Lt. to Rt.: Dave Karcher, Steve Obsbaum, Michael Blumenthal, Robert Sinskey, Emanuel Rosen and Patrick Condon.

While the JCRS was to be the mouthpiece for academic publications from the American and European societies, it was felt there was a need for a publication to report on day-to-day issues. As a result, Eurotimes was founded by Emanuel Rosen and me, with funding approved by the Finance committee. To ensure its continued success, Mr. John Henahan was appointed Editor of Eurotimes. Under his editorship, the magazine sales increased from 11,000 to 40,000 within five years and was translated into many different languages, extending its footprint into many unlikely areas of the world. His two sons Robert and Sean, remain involved in the newspaper as contributing and clinical editors respectively.

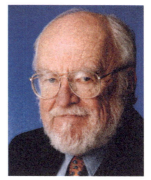

John Henahan (1928–2001)
Eurotimes Editor

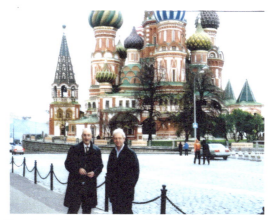

Eurotimes (Russian Edition) launched in Moscow –
P. Barry and P. Condon (ESCRS)

European Cataract Outcomes Study group – EUROQUO – Endophthalmitis Study:

Ulf Stenevi was a general ophthalmic surgeon from Gothenburg, Sweden who was a supporter of the Swedish National Cataract Register formed by Mats Lundstrom in 1992 to describe the quality outcomes in cataract surgery and was later expanded to the European Cataract Outcome Study group. This was a data based programme of cataract and implant surgery of Swedish and other European ophthalmologists and their practices. The programme was further expanded to form Euro Quo in 2008 with the delivering of the Ridley medal lecture by Dr Lundstrom in Milan in 2012.

Following his appointed as secretary to the executive in 1992 shortly after formation of the ESCRS, Stenevi participated in all the committees ensuring their full support from the executive and maintaining contact between the Board and the committees. He was a highly active member of the Program committee in setting up many of the symposia and retaining contact with the members. At a later stage, he promoted support for young ophthalmologists and was responsible for introducing E-learning to trainees. In 2003, Stenevi began his presidency of the ESCRS by launching the Endophthalmitis Study under the chairmanship of Peter Barry, which lay the grounds for the use of intracameral cefuroxime antibiotics in cataract surgery.

ESCRS Winter Refractive Conferences 1997 – Beginnings:

The first ESCRS Winter meeting was held in Madrid on the 31st of January 1997 and was the result of an executive meeting of the Congress committee attended by Emanuel Rosen, Michael Blumenthal, Philip Sourdille and myself, at the ASCRS annual conference in Seattle US in 1995.

Phillip Sourdille recalled that at that time and especially in Europe, refractive surgery was promoted almost exclusively by ophthalmic companies, and that there was no scientific society in Europe that organised meetings for colleagues interested in refractive surgery. The Winter meeting was intended to supplement the programmes of the annual congresses, and although smaller in scale, it was seen to be a good vehicle for Europe cities, which in the following years extended itself to Munich, Athens, Cannes, Barcelona, Rome and Monte Carlo. Following a meeting in Budapest, Hungary, the winter meeting expanded itself significantly into Eastern Europe ending in Istanbul, Turkey and resulting in a huge growth in membership of the society.

ESCRS Honours Harold Ridley – ESCRS Vienna 1999:

President Thomas Neuhann who came up with the idea of the Grand Medal of Merit, as "an extraordinary distinction not to be awarded every year but only where there is an outstanding personality". In recognition of the 50th Anniversary of Ridley's first IOL Implantation on the 29th Nov. 1949, Neuhann stated: "And I had the honour to present the first Grand Medal of Merit to Harold Ridley. It is unusual for an eye doctor like me myself to feel the breath of history. That was one of those rare moments".

ASCRS Honours Harold Ridley – UK 17th November 1999:

At a reception and dinner sponsored at the Swan Inn, Salisbury, Wiltshire, where Ridley and his wife lived, Dr. Spencer Thornton, President of the ASCRS made a presentation to Harold Ridley of a painting depicting a RAF fighter pilot Squadron Leader Mouse Cleavers from 601 Squadron in his Spitfire plane with a smashed cockpit canopy from gunfire sustained in active aerial combat. Present at the dinner were Ridley's two sons, David and Nick and their wives, consultant representatives from St Thomas's and Moorfields Eye Hospitals, Ms Doreen Ogg and her husband, Ian Collins from Rayner and myself and my wife Ann, deputising for Prof Thomas Neuhann on behalf of the ESCRS

The Royal College of Ophthalmologists and Rayner Intraocular Lenses – National Science Museum, London 29th November 1999:

With the 50th anniversary of the foundation of Rayner, which developed the first intraocular lens for Ridley in 1948, and the 50th anniversary of Ridley's first IOL implantation in 1949, several major events and dinners were organised to commemorate both

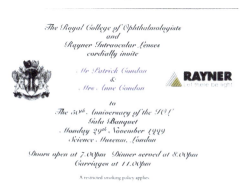

50th Anniversary of 1st Intraocular Lens Implant 1949 – Royal College of Ophthalmologists and Rayner Personal Invitation at National Science Museum, London

events. As I was friendly with Eric Arnott and several well-known ophthalmologists, including Peter Choyce and others who were known to Harold Ridley, I was personally invited to some of them. The major one was sponsored by the Royal College of Ophthalmologists in conjunction with Rayner and took place on 29th November 1999 in London in the National Science Museum, at which Harold and his wife, Elizabeth, were the guests of honour. Others attending were David and Nick Ridley, Peter Choyce and his wife Diane, Jeremy Hunt, Minister for Health at the time, Professor Svyatoslav Fyodorov from the Institute in Moscow

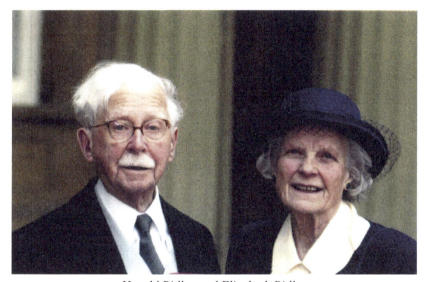

Harold Ridley and Elizabeth Ridley

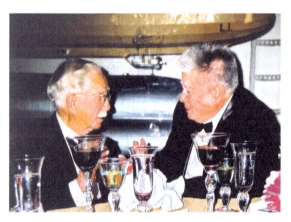

Harold Ridley and Professor Svyatoslav Fyodorov

(USSR), Ms Ann Apple, representing her father David, who was receiving hospital treatment at the time, and myself and my wife Ann, representing ESCRS President, Professor Thomas Neuhann. The occasion was marked by several speeches honouring Ridley's incredible contribution to the advancement of cataract and lens implant surgery worldwide.

Sir Harold Ridley:

Following extensive diplomatic communications including one made by the president of the ESCRS, Prof Thomas Neuhann in a letter on 4th October 1999, to the Prime Minister, Mr. Tony Blair,

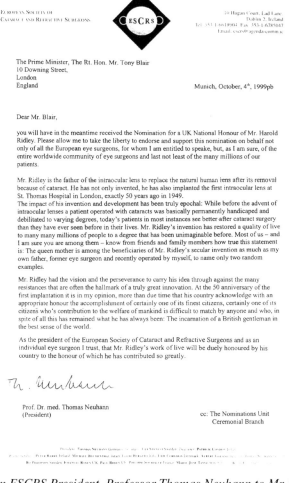

Letter from ESCRS President, Professor Thomas Neuhann to Mr. Tony Blair, UK Prime Minister, advocating Harold Ridley for a Knighthood

Ridley Receives Knighthood

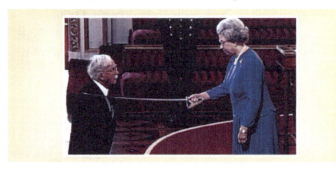

The investiture of Sir Harold Ridley by H.M. Queen Elizabeth II 9 February 2000. Photo Courtesy of David J. Apple, M.D., Charleston, South Carolina, and Ian Collins and Donald Munro, Rayner Corporation, United Kingdom.

Harold Ridley Knigted by HM Queen Elizabeth II on 9th Feb. 2000

an investiture ceremony took place in Westminster Cathedral on the 9th of Feb. 2000, in which Harold Ridley was knighted by HRM Queen Elizabeth 11.

ESCRS Awards 1999:

At the same congress in Vienna, Ulf Stenevi and I were also awarded the ESCRS Grand Medal of Merit for our services to the ESCRS. On another occasion shortly afterwards, I was also presented with the Royal College of Surgeons in Ireland College Medal from RCSI President, Professor Barry O'Donnell for teaching services to RCSI students on rotation to Waterford Regional Hospital.

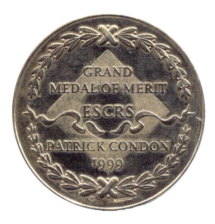

ESCRS Grand Medal of Merit

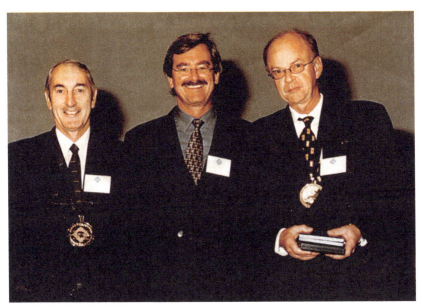

*ESCRS Grand Medal of Merit Award –
Ulf Stenevi (Sweden) and Patrick Condon*

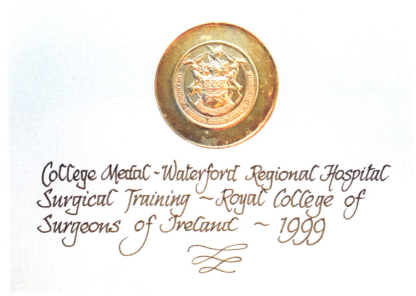

*Royal College of Surgeons of Ireland, College Medal,
Waterford University Hospital, 1999*

Resignation from the ESCRS Executive 1999:

It was at this point that I was approached by the Board and offered the position of Present of the ESCRS. With a growing teenage family, the youngest one of which had a developmental disability and was losing his sight from advancing cataracts and bilateral keratoconus, which required mmediate attention, I offered my resignation as Treasurer and Congress committee chairman to the Board but retained my membership of the Board with less personal involvement.

Chapter 20
Expansion of Regional Services – Ardkeen Hospital 1994–2000

Closure of the Eye Unit, 1994:
With the completion and handing over of the eye standalone surgical and inpatient theatre unit in 1976, Lardner and Partners, Dublin architects, secured a contract from the SEAHB to work with Swedish architects to rebuild parts of the hospital at Ardkeen with accommodation for 500 beds. As I had been involved with the architects from day one in the building of the original eye surgical unit extension, it was natural for me to continue my involvement with them over the years in future planning of the hospital to ensure the incorporation of ophthalmology facilities in the new hospital they were preparing to build. With my fellow consultant colleagues and the nursing profession, a watching brief was kept as the hospital expansion progressed. This was particularly important when it came to the planning and construction of new operating theatres for the different specialties including ophthalmology. It was also important for all consultants at this early stage to have a say in the spatial requirements and facilities for their individual specialties and the bed space allocated for patients in all the various disciplines. In fairness, the SEAHB representatives proved themselves extremely helpful and efficient in dealing with the consultants' requirements for their patients.

In October, 1994, the eye surgery extension which we occupied for 19 years, since 1976, was closed, and absorbed into the gradually expanding Central Remedial Clinic, while the remaining ward and clinic space was taken over by a growing dermatology service. Ophthalmic surgery was moved to the new general surgical block and given the complete use of one operating theatre unit and anaesthetic room to accommodate the specialized ophthalmic equipment for eye surgery, which involved the ceiling-supported operating microscope, special lighting and clean air. Facilities for minor ophthalmic procedures were accommodated in a second operating theatre, to be shared with general surgery. The transfer of ophthalmic outpatients was incorporated into a separate newly built outpatients block to be used by all specialties, but with parts reserved for Eyes and ENT in which specialised equipment and dark room facilities were provided in all rooms and came fully equipped. At first, al inpatients were accommodated in a separate eye ward with the same eye trained nursing sister in charge. As well as providing the standard nursing needs for all hospitalised patients, eye surgery patients require premedication to the operated eye in preparation for surgery quite specialised and different from other types of surgery.

"The Reduction of the Inpatient Eye Service" – Waterford Regional Hospital:

Traditionally, inpatient ophthalmic eye units in general hospitals, have always been in areas isolated from general medical and surgical patients. The reason for this being the possible danger of cross infection to vulnerable eye patients undergoing or recovering from eye surgery with the potential for developing a sight blinding sepsis condition called endophthalmitis. Also, the inpatient eyecare of emergencies and patients with eye conditions requires special nursing skills, with constant attention to detail in the avoidance of cross infection. With the initial move of the inpatient eye beds to the general ward area of the hospital, ophthalmology was at first allocated a separate ward for eye inpatients. This ward, which admitted emergencies and special treatments, was also used for the preoperative preparation of the patients' eyes before surgery and their recovery postoperatively. While initially, the eye ward functioned extremely well with a separate eye trained nursing sister and staff, it was not long before very ill general medical and surgical emergency patients, many with infections, started to occupy beds in the eye ward. This resulted in patients scheduled for eye surgery having to be cancelled on arriving for admission with their relatives. Apart from the distress to the patient, it also disrupted the normal flow of eye surgical cases leading to increasing waiting lists for surgery. Following numerous complaints to the hospital management, an effort was made to replace the admission system by centralising admissions and appointing a bed manager to process them. After several months involving multiple consultations with hospital management about the necessity for extra hospital beds for those patients requiring eye surgery or the possibility of ring fencing of the existing beds for these patients, we faced the untenable situation of being unable to function surgically within the status quo. To resolve the crisis, a request was made for a dedicated day care outpatient surgical ward, the function of which would be to prepare the patients with eyedrops prior to surgery in a clean environment adjacent to the operating theatre and to discharge them after their operation with the necessary treatment. While tacit agreement from the inpatient management system to this suggestion was acknowledged, nothing of any significance materialised, our advice falling on deaf ears.

With increasing frustration accentuated by repeated cancellation of eye patients for surgery and the constant interference in the organisation of operating lists, after 27 years of service and as the senior consultant ophthalmic surgeon, I tended my resignation to the hospital manager in August 1999 and was officially retired by the HSC on the 6th of June 2000.

The only other duty that I had to perform was to thank the extraordinarily magnificent staff that had worked with me and some with my father before me, in delivering the best possible eyecare to our patients, in particular, the late Sister Louise Ryan, and Sister Rita McGinn, and all the staff nurses, secretaries, porters and cleaning staff. On the 3rd of September 1999, an opportunity arose at a retirement party that was held in my honour at Dooley's hotel to carry out that last duty. Following a presentation to me from the staff, I in turn thanked them profusely for their selfless, dedicated, caring years of work given to both the patients and the unit.

My resignation was followed by the appointment of Mr. Stephen Beatty, FRCS. With the subsequent retirement of a second consultant, a Mr. Mark Mulhern, FRCS was then appointed. Unfortunately, for reasons unknown, both resigned their positions, transferring to UPMC Whitfield Hospital. There then followed a period in which the National Treatment Plan was requested to take over the waiting list of patients for cataract surgery from the southeast of the country, resulting in the transferring of patients to the Royal Victoria Eye and Ear Hospital cataract waiting list in Dublin. The manner in which the service had changed was heavily criticised by the public and politicians in the local media at the time.

Chapter 21
Private Eye Healthcare 2000–2018

Private Eye Healthcare 2000:
Aut Even Hospital, Kilkenny

Aut Even Hospital, owned by the religious order of nuns, the Sisters of St. John of God, was a general hospital with excellent surgical theatre facilities. With an experienced theatre and ward nursing staff and excellent anaesthetic facilities, it did not take long for the staff to adapt to the techniques of ophthalmic microsurgery. With the provision of a second-hand ENT operating microscope, phacoemulsification equipment and my own surgical instruments, I started to carry out cataract and glaucoma surgeries as well as corneal transplant operations left over from the backlog in Waterford. As the reputation of the hospital for eye surgery became more widely known, and patients were being referred from

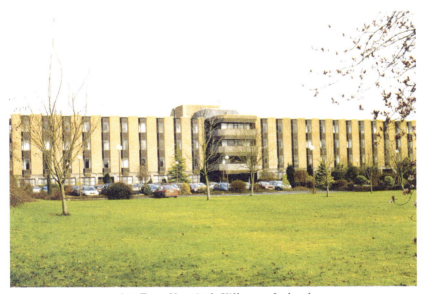

Aut Even Hospital, Kilkenny, Ireland

many parts of the country at long distances from Aut Even, the provision of adequate beds for longer stay patients on longer term treatments was a great advantage. The hospital also provided a small outpatient room equipped with eye examination equipment which allowed me to monitor the progress of patients postoperatively and those on longer term treatments.

Following my retirement from the SEAHB in 2000, I was approached by Mr. James O'Reilly who was working with a well-known colleague of mine at the Cornea-Plastic Unit and Eye Bank in Queen Victoria Hospital in East Grinstead, South UK. At the time, he was interested in returning to Ireland to work and showed an interest in joining with me in private practice. In due course, Jim O'Reilly joined me in practice in 2002, applying to Aut Even Hospital for admission rights to carry out ophthalmic surgery there and was subsequently appointed as a consultant to the hospital.

With 10 years' experience of laser refractive corrections behind me and the increasing demand for corrective surgery at the Mater Hospital laser clinic in Dublin, Mr. O'Reilly and I realised that the setting up of a laser refractive surgery unit in Kilkenny, might be an attractive proposition for the hospital and approached the sisters at Aut Even with the project. Having good relationships with the laser company, Bausch and Lomb, in Germany, at the time, we negotiated a deal in which a laser could be rented from them with servicing, which would be financed by a critical number of cases operated. Following a favoured response from management, a B+L Technolase 217 excimer laser was installed on the ground floor of the hospital with a separate access for patients. An agreement was made with the hospital to provide the eye training of nurses to take on the extra work which involved Lasik, Lasek and Photorefractive Keratectomy procedures. With the increasing interest in refractive surgery at local level in the southeast of the country, within a period of 3 years, we developed a busy laser refractive practice quickly which added considerable prestige to the hospital. In 2005, against a background of uncertainty as to the future of the hospital, the laser was relocated to Waterford where Mr. O'Reilly continued to treat patients. He then subsequently moved his practice to UPMC Whitfield, where his practice is currently located.

Libyan Experience Jan 2000:

Dr. Francis Weber, from Geneva who organised surgery courses with me at the ESCS conferences, and who had treated some government officials from Libya, suggested that we might organise similar training courses at the eye hospital in Tripoli. It appeared

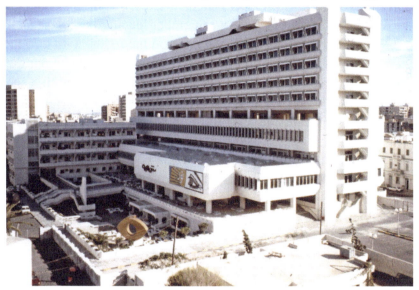

Tripoli Eye Hospital, Libia

that Libyan doctors were finding it difficult for political and financial reasons, to attend educational courses in Europe. He then subsequently received an official invitation from Prof. Dr. Khakifea T. El Bakish, Head of the Ophthalmic Libya Medical Board, to organise a small group of eye surgeons using their equipment to visit Libya. Drs. Couderc from Paris, Weber from Geneva and myself from Ireland, were all included in the group to teach cataract technique and skills development at Tripoli's new hospital in Libya. With its superb ergonomics, miniaturisation technology and portability, the OMS Diplomat instrument was chosen.

At rather short notice, I received a message from the Swiss OMS representative, informing me to be ready to

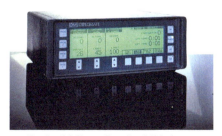

Optical Micro Surgical Diplomat Phacoemulsification Instrument

travel to Libya the first week in January 1998. No details were given to me about the travel arrangements which were kept totally secret. Without any further notice, while enjoying a post-Christmas family dinner at home, I received a phone call informing me to be at Dublin airport the following morning for the flight to Paris Orly and to check in with Aer Lingus where a boarding pass would be available for me to travel. I remember leaving the house at 10 PM on a freezing night with black ice on the roads, with a friend of ours who was also going to Paris the next day. On checking in the next morning, a boarding card was handed to me with a seat on the plane. On arrival in Orly airport, I was met by a gentleman who came up to me and after introducing me to Dr. Couderc, his wife and his young son who were coming along with him, handed me a ticket on Air France to Algeria. On arrival in Algeria, as we disembarked from the plane, we were met by Secret Service men in black suits and dark glasses in two large Mercedes saloon cars and driven across the northern African coast into Libya. During the whole journey, not a word was spoken to us, and we were treated as VIPs. On arrival in Tripoli city, we were accommodated in a large hotel overlooking the harbour with a view of the eye hospital in the distance and met up with Francis Weber and the Swiss OMS representative, who had just arrived from Geneva, and had brought the equipment needed to perform surgery at the hospital.

The following morning, we got a taxi down to the hospital which was on the harbour and went straight to the operating theatre area where we were met by Prof. Dr. Baksho and the hospital manager, who informed us that all intraocular cataract surgery had been cancelled at the hospital because of contamination of the hospitals water supply by sea water which had leaked through the foundations of the hospital, fouling up its own system. Whereas an alternate supply for the hospital was being tanked in each day from outside sources, its sanitary quality could not be guaranteed and with the possibility of the danger of post operative intraocular infection, all intraocular procedure were cancelled. A decision was then made to postpone elective surgery and to concentrate on using video and slide materials, with demonstrations using the OMS wet laboratory facilities. In general, we found the Libyan people polite and courtiers and the city of Tripoli to be extremely safe when walking around the port and harbour areas. It was subsequently explained to us that one of the reasons for the safe environment around the city was the strict enforcement of the law in relation to petty crimes, unsocial behaviour and the use of illegal substances, the philosophy for which was outlined in Muammar Gaddafi's Green Book

After a few days, we received an invitation from Colonel Gaddafi to visit his home at the secure compound in the middle of the city where he and his wife and three children were living. Following the Lockerbie bombing of a civilian aircraft over Scotland in 1988 and involved in supporting illegal organisations against imperialism in countries around the globe, Libya was regarded as a rogue nation and was being bombarded by the Americans and British regularly at night. In our meeting with him and his wife who was a teacher, while we kicked football with his sons, he expressed his gratitude to us for coming to Libya. During our conversation with him, when made aware of the water situation at the eye hospital and our disappointment at having to cancel elective surgery for Libyan patients, he suggested that we should spend some time to visit the UNESCO Heritage site of the Roman remains at Leptis Magna, which had been closed to tourists for some time.

Following 3 days of talks, viewing surgical videos and demonstrations on the equipment, our hosts arranged a night with

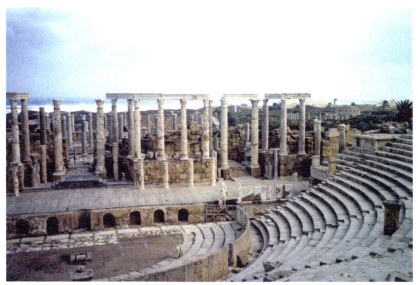

Leptis Magna Roman remains Tripoli, Libya

dinner in the desert which was incredible. When we were thinking about shortcutting our visit to go home, we received a message from Colonel Gaddafi organising a military plane to take us on a day trip to the oasis town of Sabha in the Sahara Desert in southwest Libya, close to the border with Chad, which was an active caravan centre from the 11th century. Whereas the

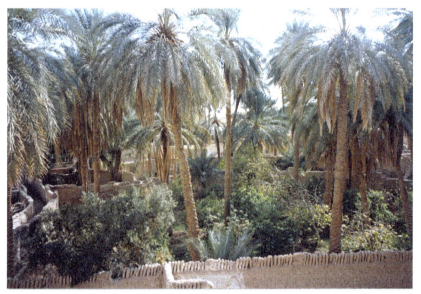

Oasis town Sabha Sahara Desert south Libya

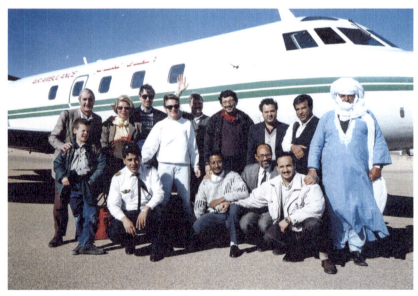

Visiting European Eye Surgery group and Libyan aircrew

centre of the town was relatively modern, the former Italian Fort Elena on a nearby hillside was used for shops, offices and houses with a large fully equipped and staffed modern hospital which we visited. The surrounding area consisted of older settlements of mud-walled dwellings and covered alleyway with a museum left by Italians, containing documents dating back thousands of years. In one of these, on a piece of parchment almost 1,000 years old, was a record of a transaction involving the selling of a palm tree in detail.

Following a week of incredible interest, we all returned safely to our homes with a great sense of warmth for the Libyan people. It was also interesting to find out retrospectively, that while we were in Libya, the meat we were eating was most probably Irish and that it could have been part of the export meat trade between Ireland and Libya which was operating from Waterford at the time.

The Eye Clinic 3 – 4 Parnell St. Waterford:

On arrival from the UK in 1973, I purchased 4, Parnell Street as a dwelling house for my family and had a small consulting office on the ground floor for seeing the odd patient privately. With a growing family of four children, I subsequently purchased the adjoining house at 3, Parnell Street extending the consulting room and using it as extra space for the family. With the move of our family to Williamstown in the '80s, the practice in Parnell St. was reorganised with the provision of extra space for more testing equipment and more technical support.

Practice Manager:

Ms Dolores Firth who was my father's secretary prior to my return to Waterford, chose to continue as secretary in my early practice ending up being permanent and practice manager. Whereas at first, she was not terribly busy, her ancillary work involved in the organisation of various meetings and the formulation of reports as the practice expanded made her an indispensable member of the practice

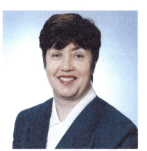

Ms Dolores Firth, Practice Manager

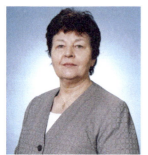

Mrs. Eileen Shannon, Applications Officer

Applications Officer:

Mrs. Eileen Shannon was appointed to ensure the day-to-day organisation of the practice and patients' records system. She was also responsible for arranging hospital admissions and discharges and further appointments.

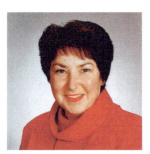

SN Mary Cummins, Technical Assistant

Technical Assistant: S/N:

Mary Cummins (OND) joined the practice with a special interest and experience in glaucoma and neuro ophthalmology. As a qualified eye trained nurse assistant and visual fields technician with an expertise in perimetry, she remained an integral member of the practice until my final retirement.

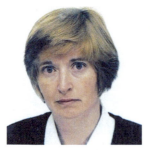

SN Marie Kinsella, Technical Assistant

Technical Assistant: S/N

Marie Kinsella (OND), joined the practice following my retirement from the SEAHB bringing extra technical assistance for patients with advanced corneal diseases, contact lens fitting in keratoconus patients and in the preoperative assessment of patients for cataract and corneal transplant surgery

Orthoptist:

Ms Beatrix Haskins trained in the UK and working with the SEAHB, also helped by seeing children with squint and vision problems many of whom required surgery in the hospital.

Beatrix Haskins, Orthoptist

Clinical Practice System Changes:

With the contacts I first made on my study tour to the US in 1970, and the ongoing continuous attendance at the major US conferences over the years there, I was always fascinated by the efficient way in which ophthalmologists organised their practices. Based on a "Fee per Item of Service" system for outpatient ophthalmic consultations, this system seemed to be the most appropriates. This was achieved using trained ophthalmic technicians to carry out history taking and the basic tests before feeding the information to the consultant ophthalmologist to make the final decision and implement treatment. Training for these technicians was made available through the Joint Commission for Allied Health Personnel in Ophthalmology (JCAHPO). Other educational facilities with higher levels of degrees were available and recognised by the American Academy of Ophthalmology (AAO).

As a regular visitor to the US for the Irish American Ophthalmological Society and other major conferences and spending some time in the company of Dr. Brennan, ex-President of the AAO, I also visited Dr. Norton Sims' practice in Fort Myers (US). His nurse technicians were using a highly efficient Cross Cylinder refraction system (Clinicon) to sight test patients for glasses, thereby shortening the rather tedious standard practice of refraction.

Following arrangements for Mrs. Marie Kinsella to work in his practice with his technical staff to learn some of their skills, we introduced an alternative way of working. With an increasing number of young patients with keratoconus and with the introduction of orthokeratology for progressive myopia in children, we upgraded our corneal topography mapping system and improved our contact lens fitting facilities.

For our cataract patients, all preoperative assessment procedures and lens formulas were brought into line with the introduction of the newer changing multifocal intraocular lens technology. As compared to the standard system in the UK and Ireland generally, the American system of outpatient ophthalmology has recently been well documented in a research paper by Harrison, R., in *Eye News* (2022) explaining the merits of the system, which with the help of the office staff and nurse technicians, I immediately implemented in my practice to supplement my time with the patients.[21]

---

21 Harrison, R.: "Working Smarter Not Harder: How to Transform Eye Care Delivery in the United Kingdom (Parts1 and 2)", Eye News Dec./Jan. Vol. 28, No.40,2022.

Chapter 22
Initiatives in Major Eye Healthcare 2006–2025

My final years in ophthalmic medical practice began to become more specialised especially in the fields of progressive myopia in children and the management of keratoconus in young adults with the use of therapeutic contact lenses.

Orthokeratology (Ortho-K): This is the term used to reshape the surface of the cornea with a contact lens in order to change the focus of the eye and is used for the correction of progressive myopia in children and young adults, a treatment called Corneal Refractive Therapy (CRT).

Myopia is associated with a continual growth in the length of the eyeball resulting in loss of distant sight and the need to wear

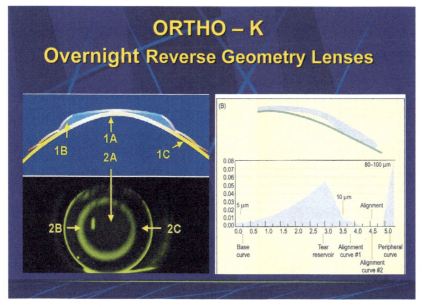

Orthokeratology Treatment for Progressive myopia

spectacles for distance. It is generally associated with physical growth and can start at any age, gradually progressing into the teenage years. In some cases, it has a hereditary background, thereby offering an opportunity for early management and prevention. Treatment consists of limiting the amount of close work especially in relation to mobile phone use and encouraging outdoor activities where long distance focusing of the eyes is used predominantly. In situations where parents are becoming increasingly concerned about the speed of progression of their child's short-sightedness, the fitting of overnight reverse geometry contact lenses which flatten the centre of the cornea not only reduces the degree of myopia but gives the child the opportunity to see better without glass during the day and hopefully reduce the stimulus for the increasing myopia.

Following visits to a busy orthokeratology clinic in San Diego for children with myopia, many with strong hereditary backgrounds, we introduced it into our practice in Parnell St.. These specialised CRT lenses were supplied to us by a firm in Phoenix, Arizona, US, and were specially made to order for each patient depending on their degree of myopia and corneal measurements. Extra special cleaning and sterilisation of the lenses were required with a major responsibility for maintenance resting on the parents. In retrospect, we found the practice of orthokeratology to be most rewarding and quite surprised that more optometrists had failed to incorporate it into their practices.

Keratoconus: Keratoconuis basically a structural defect in the internal collagen scaffolding of the cornea which occurs in young adults resulting in thinning and changing shape of its surface with considerable loss of sight from gross astigmatism. It is usually

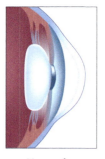

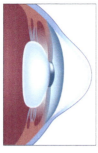

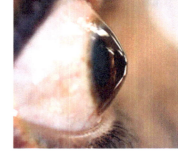

The Development of Keratoconus   *Advanced Keratoconus*

associated with allergies and eye rubbing is a factor leading to progressive loss of vision as it progresses. The problem is that it can remain undiagnosed for some period before treatment can be initiated. Treatment in the early stages consists of controlling the allergies and the tendency to rub the eyes.

Whereas spectacles can be used to improve vision initially, the use of gas-permeable contact lenses to control the excess curvature of the eye was found to be essential for reasonable sight. However, contact lens fitting on keratoconic eyes can be difficult due to the high curvature of the cornea and stability of the contact lens is hard to achieve in the eyes. In more advanced cases, the cornea may become completely intolerant to the contact lens with blood vessels growing into it from the limbus beneath the contact lens.

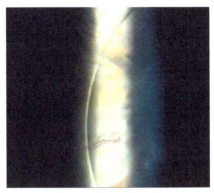

Contact lens rejection

Intra Corneal Rings (ICR's):

Intracorneal ring segments is a collective name for Intacs, Ferrara, Kera Rings and others and are small segments of inert plastic material inserted intracorneally to flatten the corneal surface and were originally used to treat myopia. I first learned about their use in keratoconus from Prof Joseph Colin who ran a special keratoconus programme at the University Hospital in Bordeaux, France and had been actively using ICR's for the treatment of keratoconus from the early 1990s. He was using a manual technique with a corkscrew type of instrument to make the channel in the cornea for the rings with good results. As there was no surgeon in the UK or Ireland using this technique and with an accumulation of several keratoconus patients with intolerance to contact lenses and almost blind without them, I referred these patients to

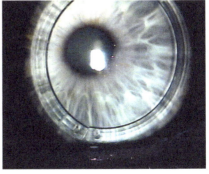

Intra Corneal Rings (ICR's)

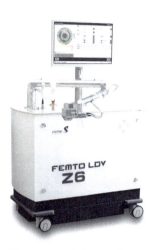

Femtosecond Laser Systems

Bordeaux for treatment using the EU medical referral scheme for treatments not available in the Republic. In 2000, Mr. Sheraz Daya, Director of the Cornea – Plastic and Eye Bank at Queen Victoria Hospital in East Grinstead, UK, started to do manual ICR's which was when I started to develop a special interest in corneal treatments. In 2004, Mr. Daya acquired a Femtosecond laser using it to make the intracorneal channels for ICR's.[22][23]

Corneal Collagen Cross-Linking (CRX):

In 1995, Professor Theo Seiler, at the Dresden University of Technology, Germany, first described the technique of increasing the tensile strength of the cornea using riboflavin vitamin and ultraviolet-Al light to stop the progression of keratoconus. He described the way in which the riboflavin acts as a photosensitising agent, while ultraviolet light improves the formation of intra and interfibrillar covalent bonds by oxidative photosensitization. This was followed in 1998, by the first clinical application of corneal cross linking being used initially for progressive Forme Fruste keratoconus.

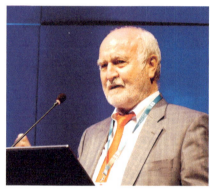

Professor Theo Seiler founder of the Institute for Refractive and Ophthalmic Surgery (IROS) Zunich

---

22 Hughes, B, Condo, P.I., and Daya, S.: "Intracorneal Ring Segments in the Management of Corneal Ectasia – A 10 Year Review". ESCRS (Barcelona), 2012.

23 Condon, P.I., Daya, S, Espinosa-Lagan, M., Espinosa, Rodrigo: "Outcomes of Collagen X- Linking in 111 eyes using "Epithelial Disruptive Technique". ASCRS, (Chicago) and ESCRS, (Milan) 2012.

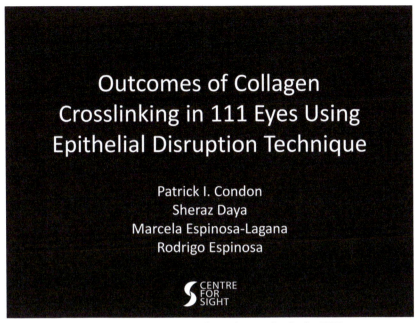

CRX Joint Presentation from Centre for Sight (UK) at ESCRS and ASCRS, 2012

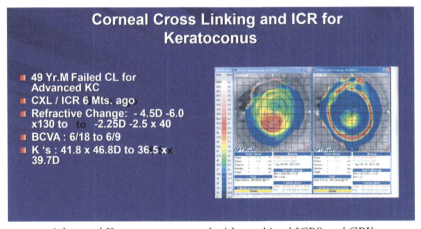

Advanced Keratoconus treated with combined ICRS and CRX – Case Report

In 2000, he moved to Zurich founding the Institute for Refractive and Ophthalmic Surgery (IROS) and started to organised courses on CXL which I began to attend. Having referred my daughter to him for PRK while working in Dresden, I invited him to Dublin where we had a meeting in the Radisson Hotel. With the unavailability of CXL in Ireland for some time, patients of mine who required CXL were referred to the Cornea-Plastic Unit and Eye

Bank at Queen Victoria Hospital at East Grinstead, UK, where Mr. Sheraz Daya, director of the unit had already introduced CXL and was beginning to combine it with ICR's. An example of this can be seen in this patient of mine in which this combination of treatment resulted in the ability to wear a standard contact lens with restoration of normal levels of vision. Failure with these treatments usually ended with the patient having to undergo a deep lamellar keratoplasty (DLK).

Final Retirement:

In 2015, Mr. John Stokes, who was appointed to the University Hospital Waterford as a paediatric ophthalmic surgeon, took over my practice and the Parnell St. premises, while I continued to consult at an office in the New Ross general practice until final complete retirement from ophthalmology in 2018.

Honoured Guest Awards

Choyce Medal Lecture. UK

2003: I was invited to give the Choyce Medal Lecture at the UKICRS meeting in Chester, UK, at which I presented our ten years of refractive surgery experience at the Mater Hospital and reported the 10 year follow-up of our patients which we subsequently published in 2007.[24]

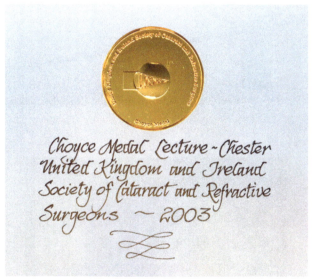

UKISCRS Choyce Medal Lecture 2003, Chester, UK

Implant and Refractive Surgery Conference, Athens

2004: I was invited to participate in the 18th Hellenic Soc. Implant and Refractive Surgery conference in Athens, and was involved in a panel discussion on Lasik with Professor Theo Seiler (Zurich), Lucio Buratto (Milan), Professor Ioannis Pallikaris (Crete) and others in which our 10-year Lasik results were discussed'.

---

24 Condon P.I., O'Keefe M, and Binder P: "Long-term Results of laser in situ keratomileusis for high myopia: Risk for Ectasia". J. Cataract Refract Surgery; 33: 583-590, 2007.

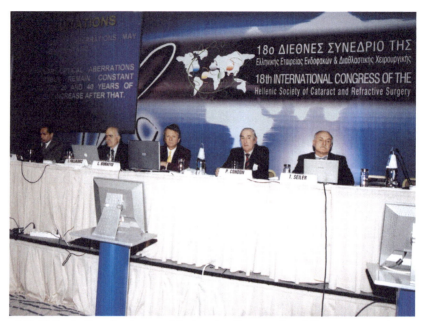

18th Hellenic Soc. Implant and Refractive Surgery Panel Discussion, Athens 2004

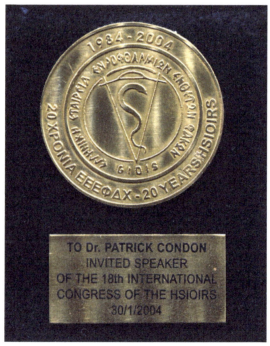

18th Hellenic Soc. Implant and Refractive Surgery, Athens 2004

ESCRS Ridley Medal Lecture . Lisbon

In **2005**: I had the great honour of giving the ESCRS Ridley Medal Lecture at the annual conference in Lisbon, Portugal, the title of which was *"Will Kerectasia be a Major Complication for Lasik in the Long" term"*.[25]

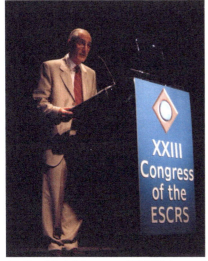
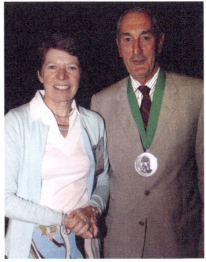

Ridley Medal Lecture, ESCRS Annual Conference, Lisbon, 2005

Medal Presented by ESCRS President Professor Marie-José Tassignon, 2005

2009: American Soc. Cataract and and Refractive Surgeons, San Francisco

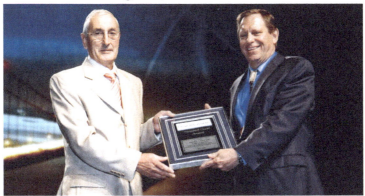

Patrick Condon receiving the 'Honoured Guest Award' from President of the ASCRS, Dr. Alan Crandall in San Francisco in 2009

---

25 Ridley Medal Lecture 2005: Condon, P.I. Jour. Cataract Refract Surg. 2006; 32:2124-2127

International Refractive Update Conference – Mater Hospital 2nd Dec. 2005:

With 20 years' experience in laser refractive surgery beginning with PRK in the late '80s extending into Lasik surgery in 1990. Many aspiring refractive surgeons were attracted to attend the meeting. Highlights of the conference were Michael O'Keefe's refractive treatment of children with refractive errors associated with severe degrees of amblyopia, and my experiences in microkeratome development.

ESCRS – UKISCRS – RAMI – "The Last Hurrah"

Following my retirement from the executive of the ESCRS in 1999, I still retain close links with members of the board and subsequent executives with the result of being nominated as chairman for some of the scientific sessions at the annual Congresses. I was also appointed to serve on judging panels especially the one allocated for electronic posters at the Annual and Winter Refractive conferences. In recognition of my long involvement over the years being a founding member of UKIOIS in 1977 and as an Council member of the EIIC (ESCRS) in 1990, I have been greatly honoured to be asked to give the following presentations in recent years:

- **2018: "My 50 Years in Ophthalmology"**
  UKISCRS Lifetime Achievement Award (UK).

- **2021: "History of Modern Refractive Surgery – A Tale of Two Centuries"**
  ESCRS Heritage Lecture (Amsterdam.) Currently on You Tube: https://youtu.be/cKOSSfwm

- **2024: "The History of Modern Cataract Surgery in Ireland"**
  Royal Academy of Medicine in Ireland Eustace Medal Lecture (University Hospital Waterford)

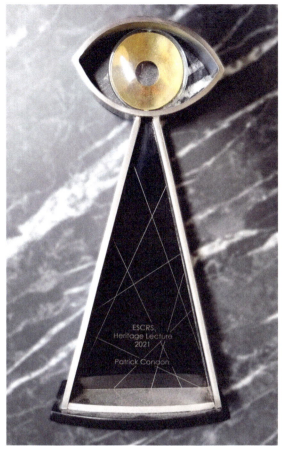

ESCR Heritage Lecture Presentation, Amsterdam 2021

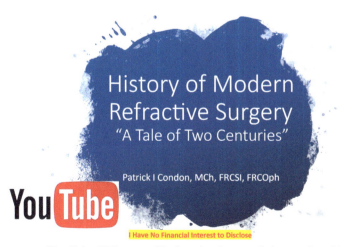

You Tube "History of Refractive Surgery" Amsterdam 2021

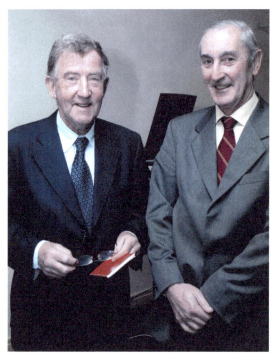

Peter Eustace (1936–2014) FRCS, Professor of Ophthalmology, University College Dublin

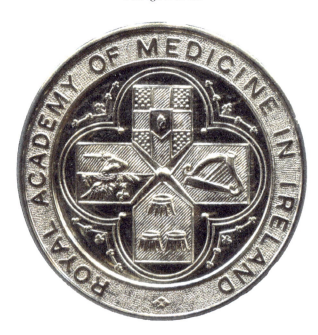

Royal Academy of Medicine in Ireland Media Lecture "The History of Modern Cataract Surgery in Ireland", University Hospital Waterford,

Royal College of Surgeons in Ireland – Fellows in Ophthalmology of International Status

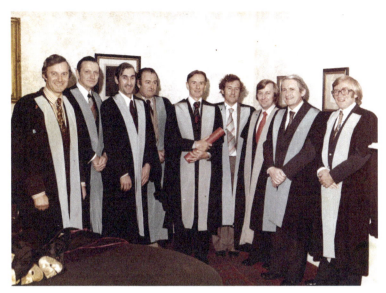

1982: Mr. Dermot Pierse, Honorary FRCS of Ireland Conferring, with from Lt. to Rt.: Eamonn Horan, Hugh O'Donoughue, Patrick Condon, Maurice Fenton, Dermot Pierse, Peter Eustace, David Mooney, Joseph Walsh, and Louis Collum.

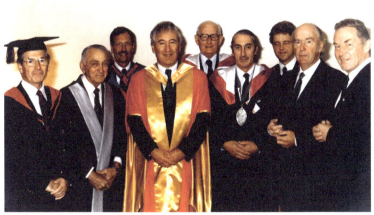

1990: Mr. Emanuel Rosen, Honorary FRCS of Ireland Conferring, with Michael Roper-Hall (UK), Teddy Epstein (South Africa), Guy Knolle (USA), Emanuel Rosen (UK), Gearoid Crookes (Ireland), Patrick Condon (Ireland), Peter Barry (Ireland), Dr. Patrick Hillary, President Ireland, Dr. Rory O'Hanlon, Minister for Health.

Lectures
- "Corneal Wound Healing with the Use of Modern Suture Materials"
- Cargill Prize Lecture 1971: Royal Eye Hospital London
- "Proliferative Retinopathy-The Jamaican Connection"
- Craig Lecture 1984: Queens University, Belfast.

Jazz at the ESCRS

My Swan Song in Ophthalmology 2008 –2017:

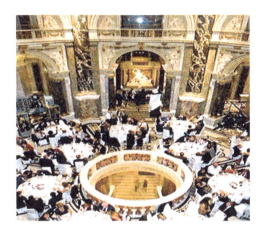

ESCRS Annual Conference Dinner Paris 2010 FFT

As a piano player since childhood, with a special interest in jazz music while attending the various ESCRS and IIIC functions, I happened to notice a delegate carrying a soprano saxophone and finally took the courage to approach him as to why he was bringing a musical instrument to a conference and never heard him play. His name was Dan Reinstein and he explained to me that when in a different city, he would always endeavour to play jazz sessions with a local group of musicians while being there. On further enquiry, Dr. Reinstein was a leading refractive surgeon working from the London Vision Clinic in Harley St, London. Apart from refractive surgery, he was an extremely experienced jazz saxophone musician who had spent some time at the Berklee College of Music, in Boston where nanny famous jazz musicians had studied. In London, Dan played regularly at the 606 Club in Chelsea and had a regular spot there. In 2007, on visiting the club to meet up with him, the band asked me to play a number with them with Dan on saxophone, which went well. Being both refractive surgeons with a common interest in playing jazz, we decided to get a group together with local musicians to provide background music at the ESCRS annual conference dinner. The first of these in Berlin in the Deutsche Bank Conference Centre in 20008, using local musicians on drums bass and a rented grand piano on a raised platform to one side of the diners, was a great success. With this setting the scene for us, and much appreciation from the executive and ESCRS members, we continued each successive year playing in Barcelona and Paris. Thomas Pfeiger, a retinal surgeon from, Austria joined us on guitar the following year in Vienna, and stayed with the group for Milan, Amsterdam, London, Barcelona, Copenhagen and Lisbon ending in 2017.

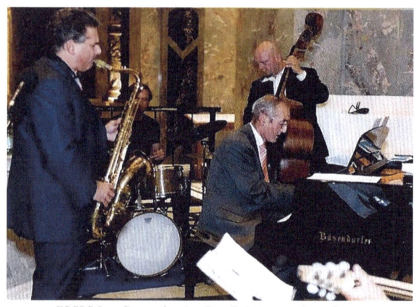

*ESCRS Jazz Group showing Dan Z. Reinstein (Saxophone),
Patrick I. Condon (Piano), with Parisian Bassist and Drummer.*

Acknowledgments

Dr. Alphie Walsh, Chief Medical Officer, Department of Health, an advocate for the delivery of ophthalmic services in Ireland, for backup support to the SEAHB (1970-97).

Much of the information in this book including many of the photographs, was provided to me by members of the Condon family, namely Elizabeth O'Driscoll, Diana Kent, Teresa McGrath, and Richard William Condon.

Appendix

Qualifications
MB, BCh, BAO (NUI), 1960, DO(Edin) 1964, MCh (NUI), 1967, FRCS (Edin.) 1967, FRCS (Lond), 1968, FRCS (Ire.), 1968, FRCOph. (Eng.), 1982.

Professional Societies
- Fellow of Royal Society of Medicine (London) – 2019 Current Fellow
- Member of the Royal Academy of Medicine in Ireland, 1976 – Current Member
- Past President of the United Kingdom and Ireland Society of Cataract and Refractive Surgeons (UKISCRS) 1994–96. Member 1977 – Current Member
- Past President of the Irish Ophthalmological Society 1988–91. Treasurer: 1984–88
- Secretary of the Irish Faculty of Ophthalmology 1978–83
- Chairman of the Congress Committee and Treasurer for the European Society of Cataract and Refractive Surgeons (ESCRS)1991 – 1999.
- International Intra-Ocular Implant Club (IIIC)1982 – Current Member

Key Publications
1. Condon, P. I., Serjeant, G.R. "Photocoagulation and diathermy in the treatment of proliferative sickle retinopathy". Br. J. Ophthalmology: 58: 650-662. 1974.
2. Condon, P. I., Gray, R., Serjeant. G.R. "Ocular findings in children with sickle cell disease in Jamaica". Br. J. Ophthalmology: 57:644-649,1974.
3. Condon, P.I.C., and Serjeant, G.R. "The eye in sickle cell disease." Jonxis Lecture-Ophthalmology Ed. Schweitzer,

N.M.J. Excerpta Medica, Amsterdam, Oxford, Princeton, Vol. 8; 147-157, 1982

4. Mulhern M, Foley-Nolan A, O'Keefe M, Condon P.I.: "Topographical Analysis of the Centration of Intrastromal Keratomileusis (Lasik) and Excimer Laser Photorefractive Keratectomy in High Myopia". Jour. Cataract and Refractive Surgery; 23: 488-494, 1997.

5. Horgan, N.H., Condon, P.I., Beaty, S.: "Refractive Lens Exchange in High Myopia: Long term Follow up". B J. Ophthalmology; 89: 670-672, 2005.

6. Condon, P.I., Terry, S.I., Falconer, H/ : "Cryptococcal eye disease", Doc. Ophthal., 44, 1:49-56,1967.

7. Condon, P.I., Brancato, R., Hayes, P., Pouliquen, Y., Sarin, K.M., Wenzel, M.: "Heparin Surfaced Modified IOL's Compared with regular PMMA IOL's in patients with Diabetes and Glaucoma – 1-year results of a Double-blind Randomised Multi-Independent Trial". European Jour. of Implant and Refr. Surg. Vol. 7, No 4, 194-202, 1996.

Books

1. Condon, P.I.: "Ocular Signs of Maternal Disorders" in Modern Ophthalmology by Prof. Arnold Sorsby Vol/. 2, 2nd Edition p. 607; Butterworth, London, 1972.

2. Condon, P.I.: "Haematological Disorders in Medical Ophthalmology" by F. Clifford Rose 1st Edition; 480-494, Chapman and Hall, London, 1976

3. Condon, P.I., Serjeant, G.R.: "Haematological Disorders" in Clinical Ophthalmology edited by Sir Stephen Miller, 1st Edition, Wright and Soames, London Chapter 21:552-561, 1987.

4. Condon, P.I. and O'Keefe, M.: "The History of Adult and Congenital Cataract Surgery in Ireland". Chapter 11; 115-132 "History and Evolution of Modern Cataract Surgery" bi Lucio Buratto and Richard Packard Fabio Group Editorial Publisher 2019.

Reading Materials
1. "A New Beginning in Sight" by Eric J. Arnott; Docwise Publications, 2005.
2. "European Society of Cataract and Refractive Surgeons – A History" Edited by Emmanuel Rosen and Peter Barry; Gill and Macmillan Publications, 2013.
3. "History and Evolution of Modern Cataract Surgery" by Lucio Buratto and Richard Packard; Fabiano Gruppo Editorial, 2019.
4. "History of Refractive Surgery" by Lucio Buratto and Richard Packard; Fabiano Gruppo Editorial, 2020
5. "Sickle Cell, Jamaica and Beyond: A Life" by Graham Serjeant; Ian Randall Publications, 2022.

The End

Index

18th Hellenic Soc. of Implant and Refractive Surgery 229–30
128 The Quay 20

A

Aesculap Meditec Mel 60 188
Agenda Communications 193–5
Agricultural Injuries 147
Agricultural Training Authority 157
A Lot to Lose Video 178–9
Alpar, Dr. John, 120
Alpha-Chymotrypsin 23
Ambulatory Day Care Surgery 125–254
American Academy of Ophthalmology (AAO) 28, 84, 129, 145, 221
American Society of Cataract and Refractive Surgeons (ASCRS) 119, 193, 200, 202–3, 226–7, 231
Apple, Dr. David 133, 205
Arnott, Eric John 48–9, 60, 119–22, 126, 132–3, 204, 242
Asante Eye Clinic, Kenya 180
Aut Even Hospital 213–14
Automated Corneal Shaper (ACS) 184
Automated Lamellar Keratoplasty (ALK) 184

B

Barraquer, Professor Jose Ignacio 23, 121, 183–4, 186, 188
Barry, Dr. Peter 131, 191, 193, 198, 201–2, 235, 242
Bascom Palmer Institute 75, 82
Bausch and Lomb 152, 156, 189, 214
Bausch and Lomb Technolase 217 189
Bigger, Dr. Samuel 135
Binkhorst, Dr. Cornelius 117–21, 190
Blumenthal, Professor Michael 67, 129, 190–1, 199–200, 202
Bromley and Farnborough Hospitals 86–7
Buggy, Paddy 158
Buratto, Dr. Lucio 186, 229, 241–2
Butterworth, Rev. Jimmy 64–5, 74, 241

C

Capsulorhexis 131
Casebeer, Dr. Charles 185
Casey, Dr. Thomas Aquinas 38, 120, 137–8
Cataract 8, 23, 25, 42, 46, 56, 74, 117, 119, 121, 124, 128, 132, 190–1, 197–8, 200–1, 229, 231–2, 234, 240–2
Catford, Dr. Gordon 120
Cavitron 124, 126, 129

Chang, Dr. Hung 119
Charing Cross Hospital 48, 119, 126
Charles J. Haughey 102–3
Children's Eye Testing Scheme 98
Chiron Technolase 116-117 189
Choyce, Dr. Peter 29, 117, 119–21, 204
Choyce Medal Lecture 229
Cleary, Dr. Philip 111–13, 131, 158
Cleary, Dr. Tom 35
Cleaver, Gordon Spencer (Mouse) 27
Clifford Rose, Dr. Frank 61, 82, 85, 241
Clongowes Wood College 35
Clonmel, Co. Tipperary 16, 20, 35, 84, 97, 156, 165–6
Clubland Youth Club 64–5, 74
Cogan, Rina 47, 164–5
College Medal 206–7
Collins, Ian 203
Collins, Michael 152, 154, 168, 172
Comhairle na nOspideal 113, 141
Community Care Services 95, 97–8, 102, 104
Condon, Dr. Patrick 51, 56, 58, 69–70, 82, 91, 101, 119, 122, 125, 128, 133, 152, 162, 168, 178, 186, 188, 192, 200–1, 207, 226, 229, 231, 235, 240–1
Condon, Dr. Richard Augustine 3, 8, 10–11, 31
Condon, Noel 163
Confederation of Optical Suppliers Ireland (COSI) 179
Congress Committee ESCRS 198–9, 202, 208, 240
Connolly Child Health Services Report (1967) 100
Contact Lens 50, 152
Corenal Cross Linking (CXL) 226–7
Corish, Mr. Brendan 107
Corneal Grafting: Book 137
Corneal Refraction Technique (CRT) 224
Corneal Transplant Service (CTS) 137–9, 167, 170
Corporate Membership 156
Creutzfeldt-Jakob disease (vCJD) 173–4
Cross Cylinder Refraction System 221
Croydon Eye Unit 36, 39, 49–50, 53
Cummins, Mary 220

D
Dallas, Dr. Neill 119
Dardenne, Dr. Ulrich 132–3
Dardis, Mary 193–4
Darrer, June 152, 168
Daviel, Jacques 1, 8

Daya, Dr. Sheraz 137, 226, 228
De La Salle College 35
Diabetic Retinopathy 175–6, 180
Digital 156
Docick, Dr. Jack 120
Doheny Eye Institute 111
Dossi, Dr. Fabiola 120
Dransfield, Helen Augusta 12–13
Drews, Dr. Robert 120, 122
Dublin Journal of Medical Science 135
Duckworth and Kent 56
Duke Elder, Sir Stewart 6, 45, 120
Dutch Intraocular Lens Implant Society 119

E
Endophthalmitis Study 201–2
European Cataract Outcomes Study group 201
European Intraocular Implant Council (EIIC) 119–20, 124, 188, 190
European Society of Cataract and Refractive Surgery (ESCRS) 190
Eurotimes 200–1
Exeter 15, 119–20, 128
Extracapsular 42, 46, 117
Eye Bank Ireland 167, 170, 172, 174
Eye Banks Association of America (EBAA) 136
Eye Donation 138
Eye Foundation 2
Eye Healthcare 21, 95, 107, 213, 223

F
Fardy, Elizabeth 170–1
Finch, Tony 167, 170
Fink, Dr. Austin 75, 83–4, 120
Firth, Dolores 219
Ford, Ernest (Rayner) 120
Freeman, Dr. Jerry 120
Friedmann, Dr. Alan 43
Fyodorov, Professor, Sylatoslav 133, 184, 204

G
Gaddafi, Muammar 217–18
Gaelic Athletic Association of Ireland (GAA) 152, 157–60, 166, 180
Galand, Dr. Albert 120
Gallenga, Dr. Enrico 120
Garvey, Michael 155
Gass, Dr. J. Donal M. 75, 82
General Practitioners 98

Gimbal, Dr. Howard 129, 131
Gimbal Institute 129
Glaucoma 109, 161–2, 164–5, 241
Gothenburg 188, 198, 201
Graefe von, Albrecht 1, 8, 11, 23, 42, 48, 73
Grand Medal of Merit 202–3, 206–7
Guided Trephine System (GTS) 140
Guinan, Larry 29–30

H
Hall, Kevin 155
Hall Lifford Hall Accountants 155
Hamilton, Larry 158
Harrington, Dr. Michael 61, 85
Harris, Brian 163, 165
Harrison, R. 221–2
Hayes, Dr. Patrick 113, 131, 241
Health Bill 88, 95
Heffernan, Christy 158
Henahan, John 200–1
Hennessy, Monica 158
Hillary, Dr. Patrick 154, 192–3, 235
Hill, Professor David 20, 61–4, 67, 69, 74, 83, 85, 87, 90, 92
Huber, Dr. Christopher 120
Human Tissue Act 137
Hunter, Dr. James 133
Huntsman, Dr. Richard 63, 69–70, 75, 86–7
Hurling Injuries 157

I
Ile a Vache Eye Clinic Haiti 181–2
Industrial and Educational committee 156–7
Ingram, Dr. Vernan 70
Institute for Refractive and Ophthalmic Surgery (IROS) 226–7
International Intraocular Implant Council (IIIC) 30, 122
International Ophthalmic Microsurgical Study Group (IOMSG) 53, 83
Intracapsular 23, 42
Intra Corneal Rings (ICR's) 225
IOGEL 127–8, 130
Irish American Ophthalmological Society 128–9, 193, 221
Irish Blood Transfusion Service (IBTS) 174
Irish College of Ophthalmologists (ICO) 191
Irish Faculty of Ophthalmology 32, 88, 240
Irish Fight for Sight (IFFS) 150–2, 154, 157, 166, 179
Irish Kidney Association (IKA) 139, 167, 180
Irish Medical Organisation 102, 114

J

Jacobi, Professor Karl 190
Jamaica 75–7, 80–3, 90–2, 240, 242
James, Dr. Geraint 61, 85
Jennings, Bernard 162–3, 166, 179, 181
Johns Hopkins Hospital 83
Joint Commission for Allied Health Personnel in Ophthalmology (JCAHPO) 221
Journal of Cataract and Refractive Surgery (JCRS) 197, 200
Joyce, James Matyn 171
Junior Doctors 52, 57, 62–3, 82

K

Kearney, Dr. Jack 120, 128
Keats, Dr. Dick 120, 131
Keeler Ophthalmics 43
Kelman, Dr. Charles 120, 124–6, 129, 132–3, 200
Kennedy, James 38, 152, 168
Keratoconus 135, 141, 172, 208, 220–1, 225–6
Keratomileusis 183–4, 188, 241
Kerr, Bobby 50, 152, 154, 158, 168
Keyhole Surgery 124
Kiewiet de Jonge award 194
Killarney 120–1, 166
Kingston 48, 75–8, 80–1, 84, 91
Kinsella, Marie 220–1
Kirwan, Nicholas 168, 171
Knolle, Dr. Guy 125, 235
Koch, Professor Douglas 200
Koch, Professor, Hans Reinhartd 133
Kohnen, Professor Thomas 200
Kraff, Dr. Manus 125
Kratz, Dr. Dick 125
Krumeich, Dr. Jorg 140, 184, 186, 188

L

Lambeth Hospital 41, 45, 61
laminated windscreen 33, 144–7
Lardner and Partners 104, 209
Late Late Show 171
Lavery, Frank 38–9, 131, 186
Lawton Smith, Dr. Joseph 82
Lehmann, Professor Hermann 69, 76–7
Lens implantation 2, 26, 29, 119, 121
Leptis Magna 217
Lewis, Dr. Ross 8, 44, 47, 86–7
Lindstrom, Dr. Richard 120, 137

Local Appointments Committee (LAC) 19–20, 88
Lost Horizons Video 157
Lundstrom, Professor Mats 201–2

M

Maloney, Dr. Bill 131
Manhattan Eye Ear and Throat Hospital 136
Marshall, Professor John 185, 194
Maumenee, Professor A. Edward 75, 83
Mayday Hospital 36, 49–50, 52–3
McAleese, Mary 154, 173, 176, 178
McCannel, Dr. Malcolm 75, 84
McCullough, Kevin 161
McGinn, S/N Rita 105, 211
McGrath, J P 152, 154, 168
McIndoe, Sir Archibald 136
Medical Director Eye Bank 173
Medical Epidemiology Unit 75–7
Medical Research Council 75–7
Menezo, Dr. Jose 120
Merck Sharp and Dohme (MSD) 156
MICRA Instruments (Micra, Titanium Ltd.) 54, 56
Minister for Health 20, 33, 100, 102, 107, 193, 204, 235
Montgomery Medal Lecture 187
Moores, Dr. Noel 46, 61, 64
Moorfields Eye Hospital 1, 5, 22, 26, 28, 62, 64, 105, 120
Mullins, Maureen 164–5
Murray, Dr. Aidan 113, 131, 162

N

National Concert Hall 193
National Council for the Blind (NBB) 155
National Irish Safety Organisation (NISO) 33, 146, 156, 166, 178
National Lottery 170
National Safety Authority of Ireland (NSAI) 160
National University of Ireland 3, 31, 35, 53, 60, 62
Neuhann, Professor Thomas 129, 131, 140, 199, 202–3, 205
Niland, Ray 159
No. Parnell Street 93, 4
Nuffield Institute for Basic Surgical Sciences 36, 38

O

Obstbaum, Dr. Stephen 200
O'Donnell, Professor Barry 206
O'Donoughue, Dr. Hugh 235
Ogg, Doreen 28, 203

O'Keefe, Professor Michael 138, 186, 188, 229, 232, 241
O'Malley, Tony 75, 85, 179
Onchocerciasis (River Blindness) 26
Optical Microsurgical Systems (OMS) 130–1, 215–16
O'Reilly, John, 171, 214
Organ Cultured Storage 139, 170
Orthokeratology 223
Oxford Congress 1, 28–9, 43, 56–7, 67

P

Packard, Dr. Richard 126, 133, 241–2
Paediatric Surgery 101
Pallikaris, Professor Ioannis 186, 188, 229
Paton, Dr. Townley 136–7
Pearce, Dr. John 122
Percival, Dr. Piers 119–20, 128, 190
Phacoemulsification 122, 124, 130–1, 215
Philipson, Professor Bo 191
Photocoagulation 91–2, 109, 240
Photorefractive Keratectomy (PRK) 214, 241
Pierse, Dr. Dermot 36, 50–1, 53–7, 59–60, 74, 83, 85, 107, 114, 120, 122, 235
Pierse, Dr. Margaret 114, 131
Pierse-Hoskins Forceps 55
Pioneers 117
PPI Adhesives, Waterford 156
Prager, Dr. Donald 122
Prendergast, Frank 158
Prendiville, Dr. Paddy 96
Proliferative Retinopathy 91, 236
Pseudomonas Pyocyaneus 86

Q

Queen Victoria Hospital 136, 214, 226, 228

R

Radial Keratotomy (RK) 184
Rayner 29, 109, 120–1, 203–4
Regional Eye Healthcare 95, 107
Reilley, Noel 103
Retinal Detachment 109
Rice, Dr. Noel 120
Rich, Dr. Walter 119–20, 128
Ridley Medal Lecture 231
Ridley, Sir Nicholas Harold Lloyd, FRS 1–2, 25–9, 31, 117–20, 122–3, 193–4, 202–6, 231

Road Blindness 143, 145
Road Traffic Act 144
Robinson, Mary 154, 168, 171
Rocky Mountains Lions Eye Bank (RMLE) 173
Roper-Hall, Dr. Michael 53, 119, 235
Rosen, Dr. Emanuel 120–1, 190–1, 194, 197–8, 200–2, 235, 242
Royal Academy of Medicine in Ireland 107, 232, 234, 240
Royal Air Force (RAF) 27, 203
Royal College of Ophthalmologists 203–4
Royal College of Surgeons 8, 36, 38, 42, 67, 69, 83, 114, 128, 137, 194, 206–7, 235
Royal Eye Hospital 1, 5–10, 40–3, 45–6, 48–9, 62–4, 85, 126, 236
Royal Eye Medical Ophthalmology Unit 61
Royal Naval Volunteer Reserve Force 12
Royal Victoria Eye and Ear Hospital 22, 44, 105, 142, 145, 148, 158, 193, 212
Ruiz, Dr. Antonio Lus 184–5
Ryan, Dr. Aidan 98
Ryan, Dr. James 20, 33
Ryan, Dr. Louis 21, 33, 96, 105, 110, 131
Ryan, Sister Louise 73, 211
Rycroft, Sir Benjamin 136

S
Safety, Health and Welfare at Work Act 146, 157
Safety Officers 179
Sail Around Ireland 163, 165
Sea-Fan 80
Seat belts 33, 144
See the Light Campaign 171
Seiler, Professor Theo 226, 229
Sellors, Dr. Patrick Holmes 36, 50–1, 59
Serjeant, Beryl 77–9
Serjeant, Professor Graham Roger, CMG 75–9, 81–2, 90–1, 240–2
Seward, Dr. Helen 133
Shannon, Eileen 220
Shearing Intraocular lens 121–2
Sheridan, Gerry 172
Sickle Cell Disease 69, 82
Sight Testing Scheme 97, 102
Sims, Dr. Norton 221
Sinskey, Dr. Robert 119, 133, 200
Sinskey Intraocular Lens 122
Sisters of Mercy - Irish Religious order 17, 181
Sorsby, Profess Arnold 8, 42–3, 61, 67, 241
Sourdille, Dr. Philip 198, 200, 202

Sport Injuries 148
Squint Services 100–1
Stenevi, Dr. Ulf 191, 201–2, 206–7
St. John and St. Elizabeth Hospital 36
St. Thomas' Hospital 1, 6, 25–6, 28, 31, 39, 41–2, 45, 63, 69, 74–5
Study Tour 74, 221
Summit Krumeich Barraquer Microkeratome (SKBM) 188
Summit Laser 186, 188

T
Taunton 15
Teagasc 157
Tempany, Dr. Kevin 181
Thornton, Dr. Spencer 125, 203
Titanium 54
Tormey, Dr. Peter 113, 131
Toughened glass 143–4, 152
Tracey, Rachel 179
Treasurer ESCRS 197–8, 208, 240
Trinity College Dublin 49
Tripoli 215–17
Trokel, Dr. Stephen 185
Troutman, Dr. Richard C. 59, 75, 83–4

U
United Kingdom and Ireland Society of Cataract and Refractive Surgery (UKIS-CRS) 132–3, 229, 232, 240
United Kingdom Intra Ocular Implant Society (UKIOIS) 119
University College Dublin 3, 31, 53, 137, 234
University Hospital of the West Indies 75–6, 78
University of West Indies 89
UPMC Whitfield 211, 214

V
Visual Field Analyser 43, 164
Visual Field Testing 109
Vitreoretinal surgery 111

W
Walsh, Dr. Alphie 44, 47, 60–1, 89, 148, 157–8, 176, 235, 239
Walsh, Tom 148, 157–8
Walter, Derek,C.Eng. M.I.E. 54
Waterford Board of Public Assistance 19, 21, 23
Waterford Clinical Society 32
Waterford Crystal 32, 96, 156, 165
Waterford Health Authority 33

Waterford Hospital Services 17
Waterford Regional Hospital 131, 155, 158, 161, 164, 170–1, 173, 200, 206, 210
Wear the Right Gear Video 159
Weber, Dr. Francis 215–16
Weiss, John 56, 131
Wellcome Trust 77
White Paper 88
Winter Refractive Conference 202
World Sight Foundation 182
Worst, Dr. Jan 117, 120, 194
Wound Healing Research 67

Y
YAG Laser (ND: YAG) 160

Z
Zeiss 43, 68, 78–9, 104, 109, 140
Zirm, Dr. Eduard 136